T0161840

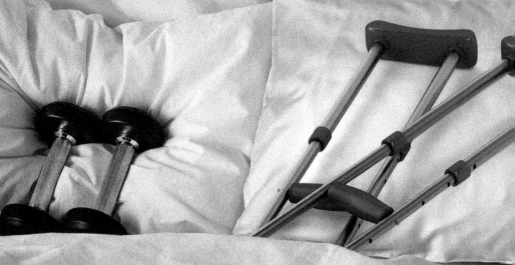

# UNPROTECTED
# SETS

# UNPROTECTED SETS

THE **NEW MODEL OF FITNESS** TO ACHIEVE LONG-TERM
RESULTS, PREVENT INJURY, AND ULTIMATELY FEEL BETTER

# SPENCER SCALZITTI, M.S., EP-C

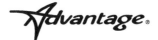

Published by Advantage, Charleston, South Carolina.
Member of Advantage Media Group.

ADVANTAGE is a registered trademark, and the Advantage colophon is a trademark of Advantage Media Group, Inc.


10 9 8 7 6 5 4 3 2 1

ISBN: 978-1-64225-311-5
LCCN: 2021920434

Cover design by David Taylor.
Layout design by Analisa Smith.

This publication is designed to provide accurate and authoritative information in regard to the subject matter covered. It is sold with the understanding that the publisher is not engaged in rendering legal, accounting, or other professional services. If legal advice or other expert assistance is required, the services of a competent professional person should be sought.

 Advantage Media Group is proud to be a part of the Tree Neutral® program. Tree Neutral offsets the number of trees consumed in the production and printing of this book by taking proactive steps such as planting trees in direct proportion to the number of trees used to print books. To learn more about Tree Neutral, please visit **www.treeneutral.com**.

Advantage Media Group is a publisher of business, self-improvement, and professional development books and online learning. We help entrepreneurs, business leaders, and professionals share their Stories, Passion, and Knowledge to help others Learn & Grow. Do you have a manuscript or book idea that you would like us to consider for publishing? Please visit **advantagefamily.com**.

*This book is dedicated to my mother, Meri Frischman and my father, Bill Scalzitti. Your constant guidance, support, and example are what set me on the path to who I am today. From our daily phone calls no matter how busy we are, to showing me how to find the positive in every situation and persevere through any setbacks, you have been the best parents any son could ask for. I will always love you and please know this book is for both of you.*

*Also to my beautiful wife Gabi—thank you for being my best friend and supporting me through this journey. You are always my biggest fan and I will always be yours.*

*To my mentors Lou Tortorello and Brad Sherman for seeing my potential early on, even before I could see it in myself, and for helping to give me the confidence needed to reach this level in my career.*

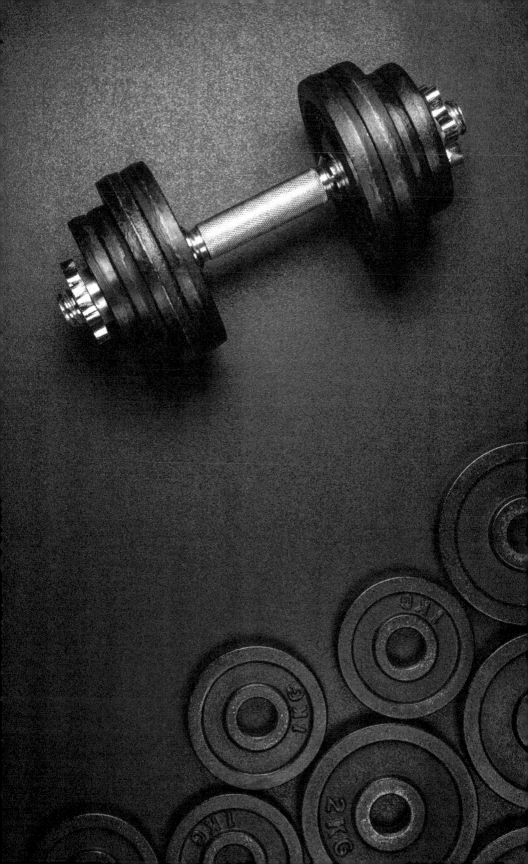

# CONTENTS

# Foreword

What if everything you believed about living a fit life wasn't true? Imagine the time wasted, the frustration of all the work and sweat, eating what you believe is the right food, and chasing a fitness dream that can never come true because the information you used to get started was based upon myths, lies, and false assumptions.

Fitness should be one of the simplest acts in the world. You eat right, do the correct workout for your age and body, rest as needed, and then reap the benefits. But fitness can also be an industry where it is easy to take advantage of the consumer because when you're struggling with your weight, how you feel, or how you look, it's easy to fall prey to the latest "secret" diet and fad workout endorsed by yet another ripped celebrity or get talked into buying just one more fitness tool because "this time, it's the only one you need to change your life!" And yet again, it fails you, ending up in the closet next to the other latest and greatest piece of crap that never delivered as promised.

I have been in this industry for almost forty-five years and have written most of the major books out there specifically on how to operate a fitness business both ethically and as a financial success. My role as the most sought-after presenter in the industry has kept me in front of fitness professionals for over a thousand workshops taught in many different countries and has allowed me to meet the best of gym operators and fitness thought leaders around the world.

But I have also met the worst. Many of the chain fitness companies, poorly managed franchises, and other fitness businesses who promise everything and ultimately do nothing but take the client's money have created a culture where the client who does want success has become hesitant and distrustful on where to turn for guidance and help. The desire for help from a willing client may be there, but we as an industry have often let this person down through simple greed and the spread of bad information. But the true professionals have never lost their faith that we could rise above our checkered past in this business.

My friend Spencer Scalzitti, a long-term professional in the industry, simply had enough with all the misinformation and client frustration. He has spent his career working with clients who have seen results and gained success through his help and guidance. His career both as a practitioner and as a medical and fitness expert working with some of the most forward-thinking medical groups in New York led him to write this book, *Unprotected Sets,* a guide for those of us over the age of thirty who want a fit life but who are tired of wasting our time and precious money on ideas and tools that simply do not work.

What will you get out of this book? If you are a seeker of a fit life, you must, at some point, be able to self-manage your own fitness path forward. This means learning how to differentiate between the social media influencer fad idea of the week and what exercises and techniques really work for you as an individual, not only to help you achieve your fitness goals but to keep you safe and healthy in the process. This is your chance to learn from someone who has spent his career working to build systems for professional medical teams to make sure all clients get the most from their fitness life in the safest manner possible, and he's using this book to share that success and proven ideas with you.

If you're the person who understands there is more to fitness than this week's quick-fix solution, Spencer will answer the big questions for you: How should I think about fitness when I am past thirty? Or forty? Or sixty and beyond? What does work and why, but more importantly, how can I spot the untruths that will set me back or possibly hurt me? How do I work with a fitness professional, and how can I tell when I've found the right one for me?

If you are a fitness professional reading this book—and I recommend every coach or gym owner do so—this book is the no-nonsense guide to have better discussions with your clients. This book gives the working professional what they need to be able to sit down with a client and deal with the questions we in the business may have forgotten are so important for them. We assume—falsely—that the consumer understands the difference between a professional coach and the ones who mislead or take advantage of the clients. This book is written for you, the true professional, to serve as a field guide to help you bridge the gap between client expectations and your personal expertise.

This is an important book. It takes a seasoned professional, one who has experience beyond the gym, to write a lifestyle guide for the rest of us who may get so frustrated at times we sometimes want to quit on our personal fitness journeys. Spencer has the experience, vision, and expertise to help us all see beyond the myths and lies we often believe that prevent us from finding success in our personal fitness journey.

After over forty years in this industry, I can say this book was a surprise for me. Finally, a book written to the average person who simply wants to feel better, look better, and get the most from living a healthy lifestyle. I hope you all enjoy reading this as much as I have, and I look forward to getting it to all my friends of a certain age who need this type of help and guidance.

**—Thomas Plummer**
Founder of the National Fitness Business Alliance and author of multiple books including *The Business of Fitness: Understanding the Financial Side of Owning a Fitness Business*

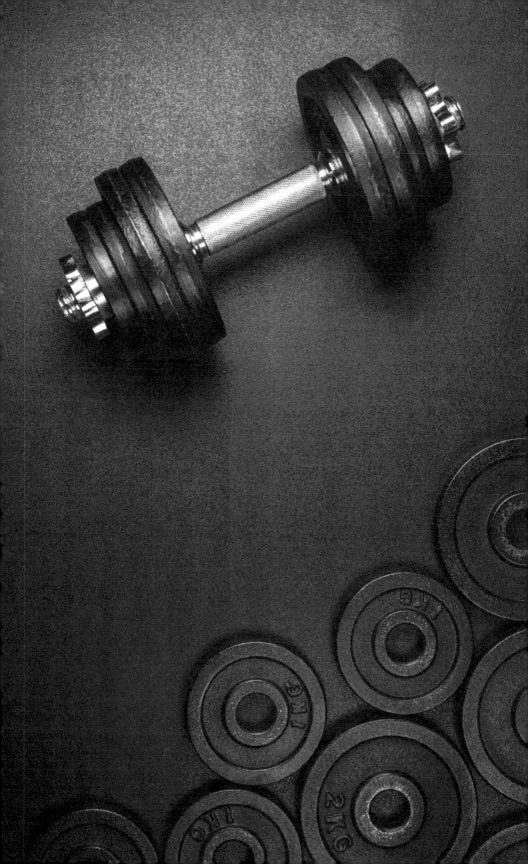

# After Unprotected Sets, Your Whole Life Is About to Change

*Many of life's failures are people who did not realize*
*how close they were to success when they gave up.*
—THOMAS ALVA EDISON

On the first day of the first semester of my exercise science under-graduate program, our professor, Dr. Jackson, started the class by asking, "Who knows how many reps and sets are needed to gain more muscle mass?" The whole class raised their hands.

Then she said, "You know what, just keep your hands raised if you *know* it's three sets of ten reps."

Half the students put their hands down, not because they knew a different answer but because they could smell the setup by the way she had stressed the word "know."

Being a cocky kid who had professional help, years of training, and fitness in my blood, I either didn't smell the setup or I just didn't care. I kept my hand straight up to make sure she noticed me. Everyone else was going to feel so dumb for putting their hands down when she validated my confidence. Instead, she looked me right in the eyes and said, "Well, you're wrong!"

She proceeded to explain how even though three sets of ten reps is the "conventional wisdom" taught in gyms, in fitness forums on the internet, in magazines, and by old-school bodybuilders, it is *far* from the truth.

Hearing this, I was filled with a mix of shock, anger, confusion, and embarrassment—but I was also intrigued. After all, I was the go-to "fitness guru" for my family and friends. I read every article in the top health magazines and fitness websites. I could list all of the ingredients in the top supplements off the top of my head. I was supposed to be the whiz kid of fitness … so how was I so wrong?

Dr. Jackson went on to explain how exercise is a compilation of many different areas of science, spanning from basic anatomy to complex biology. In the next twenty minutes of that class, my whole world was turned upside down as I discovered how much I still had to learn.

Things like how rep range could vary depending on the end goal you were looking to achieve: strength training was best achieved with less than six reps, whereas muscular endurance was twelve to twenty repetitions, and that the rest periods in between each set mattered and changed depending on the goal. Timing my rest periods had never even crossed my mind.

I learned from Dr. Jackson how recovery is as important as the training itself and that the majority of the fitness industry is either unaware or dismissive of the research and the science behind the full spectrum of exercise (which we'll discuss more later on). I began to understand that exercise is not just something you *do*, it's also something to study and practice. After everything I thought I knew, I learned there is a right way and a wrong way to exercise, that the industry's low entry bar and educational standards to work as a perceived professional are contributing to the flawed system we have

> Exercise is not just something you do, it's also something to study and practice.

today, and that fitness is a constantly evolving field. True fitness, it turns out, is a science.

I think it's important to start out by saying that even after all my years in fitness and owning a fitness business, I've found there is always more to learn. So no one should feel bad about discovering that the "conventional wisdom" of exercise may be wrong and that we all need a Dr. Jackson to come along and straighten us out. By no means do I consider myself an expert or guru like I did when I walked into that college class, but I've learned a lot—and unlearned a lot—and I believe it would be wrong not to share that knowledge, especially when I believe it has the potential to lead to real and lasting change in the industry that I love.

# Finding a Way through the Fitness Maze

The journey to a healthy lifestyle is sold to the public by the fitness industry (and the media) as a simple formula with only some infinitesimal challenges to overcome in the beginning. Over and over again, you hear, "As long as you follow the current guru's program, your journey will be a straight line to success. All you have to do is A plus B plus C—and don't give up."

Coming from a family who strongly believed in optimal wellness, I set out on my fitness quest early on and learned from a young age that it is more like a complex maze. You can follow one path for years, struggling through each turn, only to find out that it leads to a dead end and you have to start over. You might follow trusted leaders in both the fitness and healthcare communities to try to find a way out of the complexity, but maybe they end up guiding you deeper into blind alleys.

Growing from a young exercise enthusiast into an adult fitness professional, I've seen every trick, lie, and even good intention gone bad. Countless times I myself have been duped, misled, and forced to begin the journey anew, which should give you some hope that you're not alone in feeling deceived by the fitness industry. That's why I want to give you a bird's-eye view of the maze, expose the dead ends, and help you learn to navigate your way through all of the fallacies.

For starters, you can think of private company financial profit as the root cause and key motivator for creating so many new paths and dead ends throughout the fitness maze. The fitness industry is a $30 billion industry[1] and yet nearly 50 percent of people who begin an exercise program will drop out after six months.[2] Lack of success and loss of motivation are just a couple reasons why participants no longer adhere to an exercise program.[3] And although the exact injury rates

---

1   Ben Midgley, "The Six Reasons the Fitness Industry is Booming," *Forbes Magazine*, September 26, 2018, https://www.forbes.com/sites/benmidgley/2018/09/26/the-six-reasons-the-fitness-industry-is-booming/#2b0de17e506d.

2   Kylie Wilson and Darren Brookfield, "Effect of Goal Setting on Motivation and Adherence in a Six-Week Exercise Program," *International Journal of Sport and Exercise Physiology* 6 (2009): 89–100.

3   Edward M. Phillips, Jeffrey C. Schneider, and Greg R. Mercer, "Motivating Elders to Initiate and Maintain Exercise," *American Academy of Physical Medicine and Rehabilitation*, 85, no. 3 (2004): 52–57, https://doi.org/10.1016/j.apmr.2004.03.012.

of exercise may be difficult to determine,[4] it is one of the strongest driving factors that changed my own perspective regarding the current fitness model.

Furthermore, the industry has an 80 percent annual turnover rate since the average personal trainer tends to burn out quickly due to low pay, poor job training, pressure to constantly sell, and unpredictable schedules with long hours and split shifts.[5] So as exciting and nonmainstream as a career in personal training may seem, many trainers struggle with job satisfaction and burnout because of poor work-life balance, workload, and lack of autonomy.[5] These are staggering numbers and hard truths that I believe strongly hint there is something seriously awry and fundamentally flawed about the current fitness industry.

## The Movement Toward Movement

Meanwhile, the fitness industry is rapidly growing … along with our waistlines. We hear the same lesson over and over: "Exercise regularly and eat right and everything will be fine," but most people struggle to figure out what that means for them. Unfortunately, exercise today is more likely to put you at higher risk for injury than ever before.[6] And

---

4    Yaira Barranco-Ruiz, Emilio Villa-González, Antonio Martínez-Amat, and Marzo Silva-Grigoletto, "Prevalence of Injuries in Exercise Programs Based on CrossFit, Cross Training and High-Intensity Functional Training Methodologies: A Systematic Review," *Journal of Human Kinetics* 73 (2020): 251–265. https://doi.org/10.2478/hukin-2020-0006.

5    Stephanie M. Mazerolle et al., "National Athletic Trainers' Association Position Statement: Facilitating Work-Life Balance in Athletic Training Practice Settings," *Journal of Athletic Training* 53, no. 8 (2018): 796–811.

6    Nicole D. Rynecki, et al., "Injuries Sustained During High Intensity Interval Training: Are Modern Fitness Trends Contributing to Increased Injury Rates?," *The Journal of Sports Medicine and Physical Fitness* 59, no. 7 (July 2019): 1206–12, https://doi.org/10.23736/S0022-4707.19.09407-6.

we know that most diets don't work long term, yet we still recommend them. Even trying to exercise in today's world can feel more like a chore than a necessity, just another task on the daily "to do" list.

In today's world, especially if you have to juggle multiple responsibilities—family, kids, work, community involvement—it's easy to justify that "there's never enough time in the day to exercise" or to passively accept the notion that "most programs don't seem to work anyway." After a while, the risks and inconveniences of exercising may feel like they outweigh the benefits. Before long, you're asking yourself, "Why do I feel so bad when I don't exercise? Why do I keep trying? Why aren't the exercise programs working for me when they seem to work for others?" And most importantly, "What should I do now? What *can* I do now?"

Many of my clients come to me with these same struggles and make comments that may sound all too familiar:

"I can never seem to lose those last few pounds. Every time I begin a new program, I start off strong, but after a couple of weeks, I just can't keep myself motivated. The worst part is, after a few months, I put back on the weight I lost. I really feel like there's no point in even trying."

"I keep trying new products or programs with an open mind but only get disappointed again. But I want to change and improve myself, so I keep trying."

"I'm just not an exercise person. All my friends loved this trainer (or workout program), and I can't get into it. They send me new recommendations all the time, but something about them doesn't click for me. I would love to find the perfect program, but I'm starting to think it's just me that's the problem."

"Every time I exercise, I get hurt. Sometimes it's my back, or my shoulder starts acting up again, and it's just not worth the pain or risk.

I push myself to start new programs because I know I need to exercise, but it almost feels better not to exercise at all."

"I want to be able to play with my kids and be around for a long time watching them grow up, but I'm too busy to work out. Between them and work, I can't find fifteen minutes, let alone an hour a day to work out."

You are not alone in feeling this way. These perpetual problems seem to plague a majority of the general population. The good news is that it's not your fault. You have sought out the help over and over again, paid good money you will never see again, and put your trust in a system that is fundamentally flawed. There is no quick-fix solution to your health, the same way there is no quick-fix solution to these problems.

> There is no quick-fix solution to your health, the same way there is no quick-fix solution to these problems.

The years of failed workout programs, yo-yo dieting, injury reoccurrences, and that growing sense of self-doubt are not because of anything you did wrong. But here's the good news: you can be part of the solution. And that's exactly what we're going to focus on in this book—what you need to know and do to be a part of that change. There is a significant role the general population needs to play in creating a new age of fitness, beginning with understanding the flaws in the system and the cards you have been dealt.

In fact, these gaps and flaws in the fitness industry combine together in the fallacy I call "unprotected sets."

Engaging in unprotected sets can be risky and dangerous, which is why I hope *Unprotected Sets* will become your guide to a healthy, pain-free lifestyle no matter the extent of your injury history, current injuries, or the intensity of your fitness goals. Maybe you're reading this trying to figure out why fitness hasn't "worked out" for you or how you can improve at incorporating it into your life goals without getting injured. Maybe you're a member of the medical or allied medical community trying to learn what role fitness needs to play in serving your patients. Or maybe you're a fitness professional like me, trying to figure out how to explain to clients (and potential clients) what makes you different than the run-of-the-mill personal trainer filling the average gym across the country. No matter where you fall, I hope that this can become a go-to resource to change your life and the lives of others.

We'll discuss how exercise should be *reducing* one's risk for injury instead of being a risk factor for injury as found in a study by Rutgers University where the number of exercise-induced injuries increased to over fifty thousand per year, around four million in total, from 2007 to 2016, a period that also coincides with the rise in popularity of high intensity interval training (HIIT) type of workout programs.[7] We'll talk about how a lack of professional communication in the fitness and healthcare communities sets people up for failed programs and what you can do about it to take back control of your lifestyle and work toward improving your quality of life *today.*

Furthermore, we'll discuss why we continue to do what we know doesn't work, how miscommunication and misinformation are stunting our results, and how you can build the future of fitness in a way where you will finally see real change in both the industry and your body.

Through *Unprotected Sets*, I want to shed light on how and why we all tend to have an incorrect view of exercise, how the medical, allied medical, and fitness worlds have missed the mark on what it takes to prescribe a healthy lifestyle, and what—in your own mind—

---

7    Patti Verbanas, "These Trendy, Intense Workouts Increase
     Injury Risk," Futurity.org, April 9, 2019, https://www.futurity.org/
     high-intensity-interval-training-injuries-2031452-2/.

may be stopping you from achieving your goals. It's time to look seriously at how the fitness industry has continually skewed its own research for fiscal gain at your expense and why now, more than ever, we as a community are long overdue for the fitness we deserve. Once that shift in mindset resonates with you, it can guide you step by step in finding the perfect exercise program for you.

By the end of this book, I hope you'll better understand the current health and rehabilitation model, why you and so many others battle with chronic pain, how you can begin to make changes today, and, most importantly, exactly how to find the true professionals who will take you to your specific goals.

In Part 1, we'll talk about the basics of holistic health and fitness and will focus on the concepts you need to understand so you can know your role in demanding change from the fitness industry.

In Part 2, we'll answer the two most common questions asked by anybody who has embarked on an unsuccessful health and fitness journey or has battled with chronic pain and constant injuries: "Why am I always in pain?" and "If exercise is supposed to help me be healthier, why do I keep getting reinjured?"

We'll lay out a simple yet comprehensive explanation of how these questions have gone unanswered for so long and provide you with the knowledge to restore your proper health.

From there, Part 3 and Part 4 will provide specific insights and guidelines in how to find your gym, trainer, wellness programs, and start accomplishing your specific health goals.

# Enter the New Age of Fitness

With much of the health and fitness community still bombarding the public with misinformation and false promises they promote through the media, they have created a culture of unrealistic expectations. Unfortunately, this means that even those who are intentionally searching to find the right professionals or working extremely hard on programs they thought would be helpful give up on the idea that they will ever feel truly healthy.

On the bright side, some of these fitness fallacies have started to come to light, and a small group of fitness professionals have begun the difficult task of changing the industry's image. Increased professional education, groundbreaking research, new perspectives on the human body, advancements in preventative medicine, acceptance of holistic health practices, and the appearance of new sub-professions have all aided in the beginning of the new age of fitness.

Whether you are just starting your fitness journey or you're more like me and fitness has been a lifelong passion, we can work together to make changes in ourselves and in the fitness and health industry. We can stop practicing "unprotected sets" to create a better and healthier way to achieve better and healthier lives.

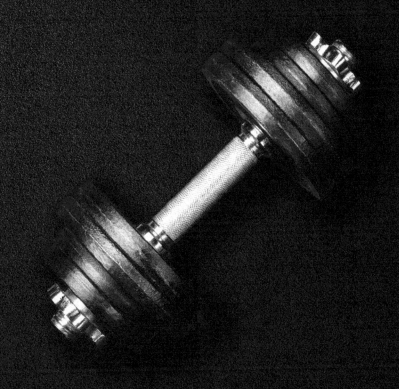

PART 1

# Why Your Body Aches, You Don't See Results, and You Avoid Workouts

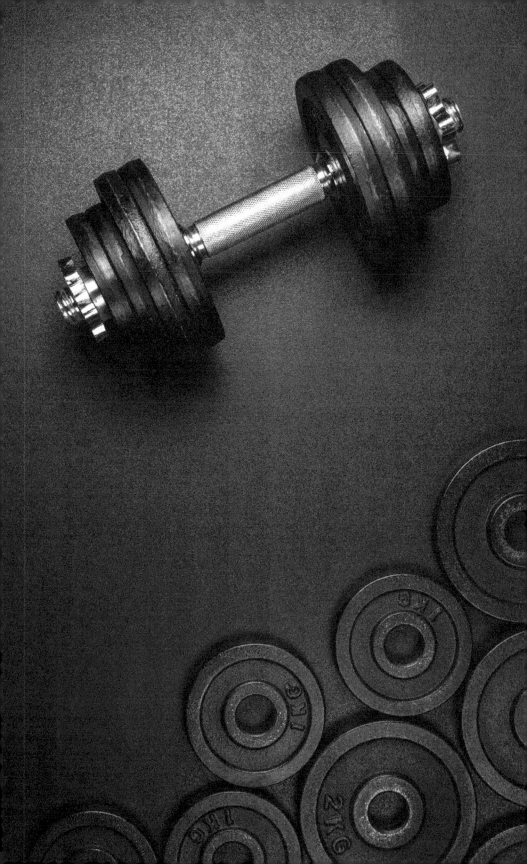

CHAPTER 1

# It Starts with a Small Spark

*Change is the law of life. And those who look only to*
*the past or present are certain to miss the future.*
—JOHN F. KENNEDY

Throughout my life, I have had several significant awakenings that led me down the path to becoming an agent of change in the fitness industry. If even one of these realizations had not happened, I'm certain I would still be promoting traditional bodybuilding methodologies. I'm a firm believer that the reason change happens so slowly in the exercise community is that even the top professionals have not experienced similar career-changing events.

One of these awakenings was the story I already shared about how Dr. Jackson turned my world upside down on the first day of my undergraduate exercise program, the revelation that I didn't know everything about exercise like I thought I did. But I probably would have been less receptive to that particular awakening if it hadn't been for a previous situation that helped me gain fitness consciousness and open my eyes to the changes that need to happen in the fitness industry.

# The Myth of "No Pain, No Gain"

Growing up, my mother was a personal trainer and wellness coach, so when I say that fitness is in my blood, I mean it pretty literally. Personal training and wellness was still a very new field back then—in fact, it was during this time that the fitness industry still believed working out before the age of fourteen could stunt a child's growth. Consequently, I began exercising with weights at the age of fourteen, and once I was around sixteen, my mom paired me with a colleague of hers so I could receive personal training from an expert.

Back then, we didn't qualify somebody for personal training based on college degrees in exercise science or by the prestige of their certifications. Fitness professionals were defined based on such subjective criteria as their physical appearance, championship titles, and word-of-mouth recommendation, which is similar to how the majority of people today *still* qualify themselves as top trainers.

My first trainer, John, was a previous bodybuilding champion and a trainer for over thirty years. He was a relatively older man, around fifty years old at the time, but still had a physique that bested many in their twenties. We trained hard a few days a week, where I would run through a gauntlet of heavy bench presses, bicep curls, decline bench sit-ups, triceps press down, back rows, and seated lateral pulldowns. We believed the conventional wisdom that three sets of ten reps at a time was the key to building size and strength. Obviously, Dr. Jackson would set me straight on that one years later.

I followed this routine strictly for the next couple of years, determined to push my body to its ultimate limits and become the best physical version of myself. Even then, I couldn't shake this painful feeling that something was wrong, mostly because of a pain in my left shoulder. But as the old saying goes, "no pain, no gain," so I pressed on—until a few weeks later when the pain was so bad I had to ask for help. Thankfully, I was directed to one of Long Island's top physical therapists.

For the next six weeks, I saw Paul (who became my first mentor) twice per week for physical therapy (PT). He did a lot of physical manipulation of my muscles, and it was a pain worse than I could have imagined, but this is what the phrase "no pain, no gain" should have actually applied to. It was like a miracle: the pain was gone, my range of motion was better, and my eyes were open. This was my first awakening because, after the manipulations, he took me to a row of exercise equipment—the same exact equipment I used in the gym— and showed me some exercises I had never seen before.

We also used a lot of very light weights, the opposite of what I was taught to do in my strength training program where the common philosophy was "the more, the better." The physical therapy felt a lot simpler than my strength training, and I often wondered if certain exercises were even doing anything because it was so contrary to what I was used to. But there was no denying the results: my shoulder was cured, and now I was ready to get back to "real" fitness.

For about three more months, I exercised like the pain never existed. I had new exercises Paul had prescribed, which I needed to do before and after my workouts, but that was a small price to pay for no shoulder pain. Then, like a bad dream, the pain started up again. Except this time it happened only when I bench pressed heavy weights, and by heavy, I mean up to 315–325 pounds. And now I felt like I had nowhere to go. My trainer was telling me to push myself through the pain, and my physical therapist said, "Just stop lifting such heavy weights."

So I found myself as a middle man between two very different ideas of what was best for my body. John never talked to Paul, and Paul never talked to John, which just left me confused about what the goal of fitness should be: bigger muscles at the risk of pain? Or living pain-free but never pushing myself? Something needed to change … but what? And what was I supposed to do about it?

# Defining Holistic Fitness

"Change" is a word that can spark excitement and controversy simultaneously. The groups that stand to benefit most from the "status quo" situation almost never want to see things evolve. And those who have everything to gain from a new beginning do all they can to push society forward. There are always intelligent arguments to both sides, which is why real change happens so slowly. But I believe we can all be agents of change for the benefit of our culture's health and fitness, and real lasting change can only happen if we are all involved.

> We can all be agents of change for the benefit of our culture's health and fitness, and real lasting change can only happen if we are all involved.

Before change can occur, you have to first know *what* needs to change, and that starts with identifying where the problems are. So before we dive into what professions and personal health practices need to be improved, we have to first recognize the current situation and get on the same page. To do that, we need to first define some concepts that will pop up over and over.

The lack of communication between my trainer, John, and my physical therapist, Paul, isn't unique to me, of course. We'll talk more about this later on, too, but the rampant noncommunication between professionals is one of several major changes that need to be made in the health and fitness space and, frankly, a big part of why the current state of health is in such disarray—bringing us to our first term: holistic.

*Holistic* is a term so overused in marketing that it's often misrepresented to the general public. In today's media, it is often linked with words such as "natural," "organic," and "alternative." Some of these trigger words can appropriately be applied in some holistic practices because holistic can also mean "all-encompassing." So to be clear, having a holistic practice doesn't mean there are only programs like meditation, reiki (energy healing), crystals, and a vegetarian diet. These are stereotypes that became synonymous with the word "holistic" simply because, early on, these types of practices could be found on some of the more popular sites promoting holistic health methods.

But in its purest form, *holistic* refers to having a 360-degree view of an individual. From the perspective of a fitness professional, this means understanding someone beyond their external aesthetics and being able to see them inside and out, what's going on in their mind, spirit, and body. Once this true meaning of holistic becomes more widely understood and accepted, I believe it should be the true approach and goal of fitness. From there, the term can also be applied to medical and wellness practices to attract clients looking for a one-stop-shop to healthcare.

I introduce holistic first because I believe it's essential for the fitness industry to reclaim its true meaning in order to promote our future vision. A holistic approach could also apply to preventative wellness or post-illness traditional healthcare. So when I refer to a community or a center, I would prefer to call it a holistic practice, but I know I'll have to wait for the mainstream media to catch up and for the stereotypes to fade away.

The second term we need to define is even more paramount to understand since it will be used at least a few hundred times throughout this book, and you probably hear it thousands of times a year: fitness.

But how exactly do you define fitness? When you hear or read the word, what picture forms in your mind?

The problem is that our media-driven culture has largely defined fitness based on what can be seen—aesthetics and athletic ability. So most people think of that sweaty person from the infomercial with the statuesque physique of a comic book superhero or the latest sports phenomenon making headlines as a first-draft pick. We hear "fitness" and immediately picture exercise models—shirtless guys with rippling abs or slender girls in revealing yoga pants. Or others hear "fitness" and immediately feel exhaustion, soreness, and are already over it before they even begin. While these images are the most common, my hope is that in the new age of fitness, they will soon only be thought of as the past.

So let's get real intellectual for a second and go straight to the dictionary. Merriam-Webster defines fitness in two ways: the first is "the quality or state of being fit," and the second, "the capacity of an organism to survive and transmit its genotype to reproductive offspring compared to competing organisms."[8] Although we need to dive further into defining what it means to be fit in the context of the industry, the first definition is self-explanatory. Fit doesn't mean being able to complete a particular push-up contest the same way that being educated doesn't necessarily require having a PhD. It's all relative.

For example, "educated" could refer to anything between having a high school diploma to a master's degree. It could mean being street-

---

8    Merriam-Webster Online, "Fitness," accessed July 3, 2021, https://www.merriam-webster.com/dictionary/fitness.

smart or having high emotional intelligence (EQ). The range is vast and falls on multiple spectrums.

The same is true for being fit. It is whatever level you need to achieve to allow yourself to live the best version of your life at every stage of your life. You don't have to conform to someone else's definition of "fit." If you don't want to run triathlons, then training like a triathlete just because such people are viewed as "very fit" would waste your time and energy. It would also be counterproductive as it would move you away from *your* real fitness goals, ruin your view of fitness, and put you at a higher risk of injury for no real reason other than trying to be like someone else.

To clarify the second definition, all it means is to be healthy enough to pass on your genetics, which means having children and thus continue the human species.[9] So if the goal of fitness is to feel good every day, move well, and reproduce, then why is it so normal and accepted for us to think of abs, bodybuilders, triathletes, models, and professional athletes instead? If you haven't already guessed it, the answer is *marketing*. It's hard to sell a program when you're telling somebody that they need to quickly get up a flight of stairs or move without pain to be considered fit. It's far easier to sell a program saying, "Don't you want to look like *this*?" and point to a picture of the smiling model.

Beyond that, it's much easier to fearmonger and play with people's emotions on sensitive topics like weight gain and societal approval. Thus came the popularity of bodybuilders, beach physiques, and weight-loss gimmicks. It's just a more expedient way to make money. We'll revisit this idea of aesthetics-selling more in depth later

9    Peter D. Gluckman and Carl T. Bergstrom, "Evolutionary Biology within Medicine: A Perspective of Growing Value," *BMJ*, (December 2011): 343: d7671, https://doi.org/10.1136/bmj.d7671; Thomas B. Kirkwood and Steven N. Austad, "Why Do We Age?," *Nature* 408 (2000): 233–8, https://doi.org/10.1038/35041682.

on, but nothing else will make sense if you can't start to question the mythical version of holistic fitness and define it in a healthier context.

Now, there are a couple other things we need to define so you can track along with me. First, you need to understand the difference between the terms "health community" and "allied health community." When I refer to health professionals, I'm primarily talking about doctors, but allied health professionals can include a large scope of different types of professionals and specialists. But to keep things simple, I'll just define the primary ones that we'll refer to throughout the book and overlap the most with the fitness industry:

- Physical therapists (PT), which could include specialists in both rehabilitation therapy (after surgery) or prehabilitation therapy (before surgery),

- Occupational therapists (OT), who focus more on helping patients with being able to handle everyday living skills,

- Chiropractors (chiros), who focus on the musculoskeletal system in their patients, and

- Nutritionists, who will focus on helping patients identify their specific nutrition needs based on a range of individual factors. A level beyond this is a registered dietician (RD), which is typically an individual who has more credentials and education than the average nutritionist.

There are others, of course, but these tend to be the most recognized in the current state of the fitness industry who can help play a role in one's holistic fitness journey.

Another definition we need to get out of the way now—and probably one of the biggest misunderstandings that I see in the public—is the difference between a fitness professional (FP) and a personal trainer. Many times, I see these terms used interchangeably, but they are *not* the same thing.

A lot of the time, the term "fitness professional" gets used as a blanket term to encompass everything from a part-time personal trainer at a gym, the person leading a spin class, or even a certified exercise physiologist (EP).

A personal trainer typically only focuses on the exercise angle of things, particularly in the context of a specific workout program they represent and utilize with all of their clients, regardless of the individual's needs. Don't get me wrong—I'm not saying that personal trainers don't care about their clients. Remember, my mom was one, and I can vouch that she really cared for her clients, but a lot has changed since then. At the end of the day, your average personal trainer simply has not been trained to help their clients from a holistic perspective.

On the other hand, I define a fitness professional as someone who focuses on coaching an individual by knowing them on a personal level. This includes understanding their unique health goals and needs and how they should align with their fitness plan while also considering their mental and social health. In other words, the FP is looking at the *whole* person, their *holistic* health. An FP also has more formal education in health and fitness than your average personal trainer, which I'll explain in more detail later on. So while there may be components of personal training that fit into the FP's plan for their client, it would be wrong to assume that the two are the same thing.

The same could be said about an exercise physiologist, which is a step beyond an FP because of the level of certification and training they have achieved. In fact, an EP should have a bachelor's degree and some specialized certifications—at bare minimum—and eventually perhaps a master's degree. So there may be overlaps between these three types, but each of them is approaching exercise from a different perspective and with a different goal. Don't worry—we'll talk about this more later on when we discuss some keys to finding the right FP and gym for you, but for now, knowing these basic differences should be enough.

## Beach Bodies Create Broken Bodies

Later on, we'll outline how to navigate your way through today's fitness industry because, let's face it, it's not going to change overnight, and there is no "one size fits all" solution if we are going to move toward a holistic approach. After all, we have an industry with the potential to produce results and solve many of the country's health problems, but it has turned into a field of "quick fixes" and money-making schemes. The industry promises happiness and claims to deliver it through aesthetics.

> We have an industry with the potential to produce results and solve many of the country's health problems, but it has turned into a field of "quick fixes" and money-making schemes.

Therefore, the visual appeal of perfect abs and sculpted arms has taken precedence over what I would consider more important goals like disease prevention or a lifetime of pain-free movement. Smiling faces with thin waists are paraded at the head of every fitness campaign, sending the not-too-subtle message that "with our program (or facility), you will gain the same results!"

Besides this being statistically untrue, there is no mention of the people who have dropped out due to pain or injury. There is no discussion about how the person behind that smiling face is doing six months after completing the program nor any mention of the extra work they had to put in *outside* of the program to achieve those photogenic results in the first place.

This altered version of reality, combined with the "no pain, no gain" thinking, helps to reinforce and perpetuate two fundamentally incorrect assumptions. The first is that if somebody is lean and muscular, they must be fit. The second is that the person who can work the hardest, jump the highest, or do the most repetitions is also the most fit person. These dangerous and erroneous assumptions do not take into account that same person's constantly aching shoulder pain, knee pain while walking up stairs, or the possibility of a double knee replacement by age fifty-five. Maybe you can bench 225 pounds, but if you're constantly in and out of physical therapy for years on end, are you really fit?

## Change Starts with Individuals

So what does a real fitness program look and feel like? How many days a week should you exercise? If the goal isn't supposed to be aesthetics, then how can you know when you're fit?

The answers are simple. As long as you don't have an underlying health condition that would change your guidelines for exercise[10] and as long as you are under the care and supervision of a true fitness professional, your fitness program can look and feel however you want. That may be a hard concept for people to wrap their heads around because the next thought is, "Well, if it's however I want, then I want it to be sitting on my couch watching television, and I want it to feel like a dream because I'd rather be sleeping."

---

10  Geoffrey E. Moore, J. Larry Durstine, and Patricia L. Painter, *ASCSM's Exercise Management for Persons with Chronic Diseases and Disabilities*, 3rd ed. (Champaign, IL: Human Kinetics, 2009).

But this is where it's important to work with an FP who really knows you well and can make the appropriate recommendations designed just for *you*. Change has to begin on an individual level, which requires putting in real time and work to figure out what that looks like for you over the long term, not the "quick fix" that your average gym or fitness facility is selling.

From my perspective, the current model of fitness is based solely on aesthetics and achieving an ideal weight, which is reflective of a quantity over quality model. Hear me loud and clear: bodybuilding, weight loss training, or aesthetics programs are *not* the enemy, but they are also not the "end-all be-all" of fitness. Demonizing any one modality of fitness is not helpful, as there is a place for all types of fitness, and each of these can play an appropriate role in an individualized holistic fitness plan.

The misconception comes into play when there is nobody to explain the damage that may be done as a consequence of "unprotected sets." If a person is warned by an FP or personal trainer that the bicep curls they are doing might restrict their shoulder mobility and cause future neck or elbow pain, then it would be their own responsibility and fault for ignoring that advice. However, the general public is not informed about the realities in most fitness programs, leaving the responsibility on the shoulders of the fitness industry for its lack of transparency and accountability to the public.

Even if you were to embark purely on an aesthetics goal, the fitness professional's other job is to find out where on the spectrum of function and movement you fall. This means a full movement screening and specific muscle testing should be conducted first.

For example, if you have back pain, poor biomechanics of the hip, or improper dynamic motor control at your pelvis, your fitness professional should find that out in a screening/assessment. Then their programming for you should not only take out those loaded back squats you have done for years, but they should also have an arsenal of regressed exercises for you to master first.

These exercises would probably include things like mobility techniques, stabilization strategies, muscle activation procedures, neuromuscular patterning drills, and other tools that would correct your dysfunctions. These types of assessments and treatment protocols can make a program run much longer than originally thought, but if not executed properly, it can set the person up for future injury and pain. Thus, the current fitness community is practicing a model that struggles to create the results that it has promised and that the public deserves.

I know this is a lot to process, and I've had the advantage of spending a lot of time learning and experiencing these ideas firsthand. So while there is no "quick fix" to the system, maybe I can save you some time from having to figure things out the hard way. In the following chapters, I promise we'll break down each of these concepts: the problems in the system and what needs to change from handling injuries to better understanding your personal motivations for better fitness. We'll start at a high level, understanding the current system and work our way down to understanding yourself and your choices. Because real change has to start with *you*.

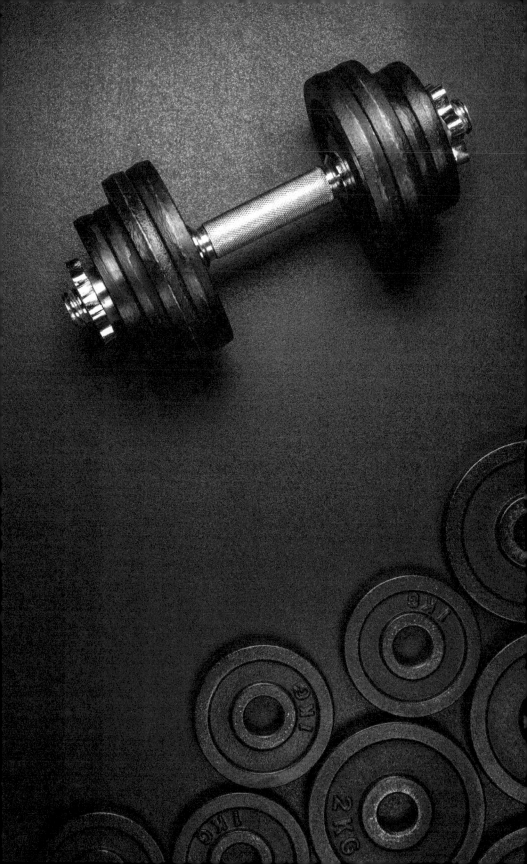

# CHAPTER 2

# All Pain, No Gain

*The definition of insanity is doing the same thing over
and over again expecting different results.*
—ALBERT EINSTEIN

We need to go back now to the story I started in the last chapter. As you might recall, I felt stuck between two differing views of what was best for my fitness, and I wasn't sure what to do next. So I asked John, my personal trainer, if he would speak to Paul, my physical therapist, and I asked Paul to talk to John.

I did not know at the time, but it turns out that kind of communication was very uncommon practice. In fact, it still kind of is uncommon. No professional wants to step on the toes of another and say, "I think you're wrong." What I saw simply as working together, they would see as disrespect and stepping out of their own professional scope of practice. All I wanted was the perfect game plan sculpted by the two professionals I trusted. But because they were stuck in their silos, because there was no holistic approach, they couldn't help my specific situation and goals become a reality. So for the next few years, I continued to exercise for muscular size and strength when the pain was minimal and returned to physical therapy each time the pain became unbearable.

It's important to understand I'm not aiming to degrade or place blame on any one field or subsection of that field. Still, each section of the current healthcare and allied healthcare models plays a role in why the current state of America's health is in such disarray—ranging from orthopedic practices to today's physical therapy model. The emphasis made during the discussions of each field often results in a lack of collaboration and communication between them. So I believe there is no one specific link in the chain that is more at fault than the other, but that the whole chain itself is broken. Understanding this first is the key to taking back control over your own wellbeing.

# Whose Fault Is It Anyway?

We seem naturally wired as humans to look for something—or someone—to blame. For example, it's easy to blame that box you just picked up as the reason your back hurts. When there is no obvious "culprit," though, or if you've done all the right things like changed your diet, started a workout regimen, seen the doctor, and so on, then you might eventually place personal blame on yourself to shift away from it possibly being anybody else's fault: "I must have moved wrong. I really should have bent down using my legs more. Maybe it's just the way I'm made. I've been too lazy and should be working out more." Or the classic: "The box was too heavy, but I thought I could lift it. No one to blame but me."

While there's nothing inherently wrong with looking at your own actions and finding where you need to improve, the real problem here is that it just *might* be everybody else's fault, or to put it another way, we all share the fault as a culture. You can't remember it, but you moved amazingly well when you were a baby. We are born with the perfect mechanics for crawling, squatting, deadlifting, and rolling over. Some fitness companies even form their programs around how to get adults to move more like infants, to unlearn all the unhealthy mechanics we've picked up over time. In fact, research has even been conducted studying the biomechanics of how children run to help adult runners learn better running form, or again, unlearn bad form that has been picked up over time.[11]

If you've ever watched a baby pick up or play with a toy on the ground, maybe you've noticed how their butt sinks right to the ground, their knees easily fold up toward their chest and they can sit there playing for hours. Now, as an adult, try to play with a toy on the ground while keeping both feet flat on the floor. Better yet, challenge your friends to get down on all fours and crawl across a room. You could bet your annual salary that most of them won't make it, and if they do, they will collapse on the ground writhing in pain.

There are dozens of books in the fitness and movement industry that discuss the theories behind movement inefficiency. They discuss how to improve these movement patterns and how to reteach this type of "motor learning."[12] You can read every book on the subject, but the questions will still remain as to why you never knew about this before,

11    Benedicte Schepens, Patrick A. Willems, and Giovanni Alfredo Cavagna, "The Mechanics of Running in Children," *Journal of Physiology* 509, no. 3 (1998): 927–940, https://doi.org/10.1111/j.1469-7793.1998.927bm.x

12    Moshe Feldenkrais, *Awareness Through Movement: Easy-to-Do Health Exercises to Improve Your Posture, Vision, Imagination, and Personal Awareness*, illustrated ed. (New York: Harper Collins, 2009); Richard Schmidt and Timothy Donald Lee, *Motor Learning and Performance*, 6th ed. (Champaign, IL, Human Kinetics, 2019); Stuart McGill, *Ultimate Back Fitness and Performance*, 6th ed. (Waterloo, Canada, Backfit-pro, 2017).

or if you did, why did you decide to settle for this level of discomfort as what life is supposed to be like "after a certain age"? Where did it all first start going wrong? And who should be helping you set it right?

Let's begin by visiting one of the more "umbrella" explanations for recurring pain and injury, which is focused on the time we spend physically inactive, particularly sitting, and the negative results that follow.[13] It started back when your parents told you to stop playing and sit down for dinner. It continued when the school system told you to sit and focus for eight hours straight for over a decade. As we grow, we start to spend more and more time sitting, which is partially to blame for how our mechanics start to change, but then the blame shifts to the workplace.

From a functional movement standpoint, our days began to look like this: we wake up and *sit* in the kitchen as we have our coffee and eat breakfast. We *sit* in our car and drive to work, where we *sit* from nine to five, then drive home (*sitting* in our car again) and then *sit* and eat dinner. We finish up the day with more *sitting* in front of the television or even in a chair and reading our favorite book, and then it's time to do it all over again the next day. Instead of only sitting for eight hours straight for a decade during your school-age years, it turns into eight hours straight of sitting for your *entire* life. Obviously, this is assuming you have a typical desk job. Some people get more physical activity in their work, but not on the scale that it used to happen.

Simply put, if you're forty-three years old and you stopped playing like a baby at three, you've been sitting or lying down (sleeping) for the majority of each day of those forty years. That's 350,400 hours, or 21,024,000 minutes, of sitting and lying down. So is it really any wonder why we don't move like we used to?

---

13   Kelly Starrett, *Deskbound: Standing Up in a Sitting World*, 1st ed. (Las Vegas: Victory Belt Publishing, 2016).

So the first answer to the question of why you are always getting injured is that the current lifestyle we engage in is actually setting you up for injury. When we sit, we tighten and shorten certain muscle groups while lengthening and weakening the opposing muscle groups.[14] When we stand up, these changes in the muscle tissue do not quickly revert back to their natural lengths but can take hours or days of moving again to get them back to where they should be or even large

> So the first answer to the question of why you are always getting injured is that the current lifestyle we engage in is actually setting you up for injury.

chunks of time stretching to correct a few hours of sitting. The body is very efficient, and once it recognizes a position you like to engage in, it lays down more tissue in the form of fascia[15] to strengthen your body's ability to stay in that position for long periods of time.

If you've never heard of fascia, don't be too hard on yourself. I'd never heard about it either until after I got my degree. In exercise, there's a ton of talk about muscles—abs, glutes, deltoids, biceps—so people tend to know about those. Especially if you've ever participated in any kind of HIIT program, a topic we'll delve into later, there's *lots* of muscle talk: "This will target your quads, this will target your pecs," and so on.

One of the issues I take with these programs is that their focus on muscles doesn't take a holistic view of the body. Some scientists even propose that these muscles don't actually exist in the way they've

---

14  Starrett, *Deskbound*.

15  David Lesondak, *Fascia: What It Is and Why It Matters*, 1st ed. (Pencaitland, Scotland: Handspring Publishing Ltd., 2017); Thomas Myers, *Anatomy Trains: Myofascial Meridians for Manual and Movement Therapists*, 3rd ed. (London: Churchill Livingstone, 2014).

been traditionally taught, that they are instead all connected, but that we've divided them up more for practical reasons in the same way that we draw state lines on a map.

One of the reasons I mention this is because it's entirely possible that the pain you feel in one muscle could actually be caused from a movement in a different part of your body because it's all connected. For example, if you pull down on the bottom of your shirt, it's going to also pull down the collar and the fabric around your shoulders. And that's where fascia comes in.

Without getting too lost in the science, fascia is thin tissue that encases and connects every part of your body, organs, muscles, bones, nerves, blood vessels—you get the idea. Now, even though it's not a perfect analogy, think of fascia as plastic and muscles as elastic. Muscles will rebound and stretch back like elastic, but the fascia tissues will behave more like plastic. Imagine you pull a plastic bag from each end and then set it down to watch how long it takes to go back to its original shape—if it ever does. You've got a better idea then of how long it takes for fascia to get back "into shape."

It sounds like an adverse reaction by the body, but this is actually how brilliant nature truly is. Muscles can't stay in a position very long without getting tired, so it needs the fascia to support it. Think of it like this: the average head weighs seven to nine pounds, so what would hold a nine-pound bowling ball for longer? A bag made of elastic? Or a bag made of thick plastic? The elastic bag would immediately fall prey to gravity and drop the ball to the ground, even tearing the elastic, while the plastic bag would be able to hold it much longer before tearing.

But just as the fascia is strong in holding you in the seated position or keeping your head from collapsing while you push it forward to read emails on your computer, it's just as hard to break down, manipulate, and change when you have spent too many hours—or decades—in a particular position. Now, I admit that's an extreme oversimplification of the process the body undergoes to keep you in whatever position you want it to be in again, but I also don't want to bore you to death. And there are some really amazing books on the topic of how to move well again,[16] but there's a lot more that goes into why you may always be feeling pain.

Now, this discussion focused only on what set you up for pain which proposes the question as to why haven't you heard this before? Maybe it is because traditional/conventional education regarding injury and recovery only focuses on how to *treat* it—a reactive approach—as opposed to prevention—a proactive approach.

Also, you haven't heard of this because it just simply isn't taught on a large scale, so you can't know what you don't know. In a sense, it's "easier" to think of muscles and locations of pain, but that takes a limited view of both the body and the potential problem. In short, this is something that the healthcare community technically understands and should take into consideration with injuries, yet my experience has been that it enters the injury conversation far less than it should. And frankly, most people in the fitness industry are not taught about this because exercise has traditionally focused on muscles rather than considering how they are connected.

## Why Does This Keep Happening?

This leads to the next question we need to discuss: When you go for help after an injury—or after you've had the surgery that was supposed to correct the injury—why do you still seem to get injured again and again?

---

16    Kelly Starrett, *Becoming a Supple Leopard: The Ultimate Guide to Resolving Pain, Preventing Injury, and Optimizing Athletic Performance*, 2nd ed. (Las Vegas: Victory Belt Publishing, 2015); Gray Cook, *Athletic Body in Balance: Optimal Movement Skills and Conditioning for Performance*, 1st ed. (Champaign, IL: Human Kinetics, 2003).

Let's paint a picture, one that might sound and feel very familiar to you. Imagine it's a cold winter morning. You roll over and look at the alarm clock only to realize you've overslept. Don't worry ... this is a safe space, you can admit it here. Anyway, you jump out of bed, get dressed in haste, and on the way out the door, you reach down to pick up your bag, only to throw out your back again.

This is the third time in two years, and you cannot spend *another* day on the couch. You've seen the doctor before, you've been to physical therapy, visited the chiropractor quarterly, and you even work out two to three times a week. Maybe you even switched from your fitness DVD that promised you a stronger core to a personal trainer who promised you the same thing but now under their supervision to help you with better form or new techniques. So why is this happening again?

The first time this happened, your doctor said, "It's a herniated disc, but the physical therapy will help." And it did. When you left PT, you felt so much better, so how could you possibly still be dealing with injuries? Many people experience this type of scenario throughout their lives or know somebody close to them who has been through a similar situation.

This scenario could apply to any pain, not just back problems. Maybe it is your constant shoulder pain, neck pain, or knee pain ... you fill in the blank. It could even be the first time you have experienced back pain, but two years ago, it was your wrist or ankle. During that time, you sought out help instead of ignoring the problem, and every professional you saw did their job to their fullest extent. They even came highly recommended by a friend or colleague, leaving you with the only place left to go: self-diagnosis.

Questions start to occupy your mind like "Is it my shoes? Do I sit too much? Is it a neurological problem?" or the most extreme: "Is this a sign something more serious is going on here?" While these are important questions to ask and always worth delving into if the pain is chronic or recurring, let's first take a step back and look at the rehabilitation system as a whole.

When an injury occurs, whether from an exercise program—or lack thereof—the first stop is typically the doctor's office. This may be an internist or straight to a specialist, that is, a health professional with a specialized focus on the part of the body that appears to be giving you grief. After a brief visit, a diagnosis is made, and you're sent for further testing, which can range from muscle tests to MRIs so that a more conclusive diagnosis can be given. If there happens to be more severe damage like a torn ligament or osteoarthritis, cortisone shots, or even surgery may be recommended. Rehabilitation is the most common recommendation for post-surgery or even for lesser injuries that did not require more extreme measures.

The next stop is your doctor-recommended physical therapy center. The field of PT is a vastly growing field that has done amazing work in terms of injury rehabilitation and pain relief. Like the rest of the medical community, though, many of the tests and treatment protocols are not always guided by what is best for the patient on an individual basis, but by insurance companies and *their* protocols, what is covered, when it can be covered, and so on. If you enter a PT office with shoulder pain, an examination of the shoulder function will be administered, followed by treatment at that specific joint. This approach is effective for pain relief, especially in a system where the therapist needs to see many patients per day.

Since insurance pays per visit and only allows a certain number of visits that they will cover, the therapist must show as much improvement to the current diagnosis as quickly as possible. New research and new approaches to pain management which looks more globally (or holistically) for the root cause of issues challenges the traditional version of rehabilitation and may eventually cause a radical change in how physical therapists perform both assessments and treatment. But we'll explore this topic more in Part 2.

Traditionally, the medical field has taken a local approach to diagnosis, meaning you go to the doctor and say, "Hey, my left shoulder hurts." They examine it, give a diagnosis, recommend a remedy that will hopefully fix the issue, and then you're sent on your way. But to go back to the shirt example, the tightness you feel in your shoulders may be caused by a "pull" happening elsewhere within the body. A global approach would take this into consideration.

## Life After Insurance

As I mentioned earlier, many of the medical decisions and advice are directed more by insurance providers than what is best for the patient, so the question now becomes what do you do if your allotted amount of insurance visits runs out? If you have previously engaged in an exercise program at a local gym, group fitness classes, or an at-home exercise program, it may be "back to the same routine" for you. If the injury happened during an exercise program or around the time an exercise program increased its intensity, this may steer you away from returning to the same program. With minimal guidance given to the general public of what qualifies as an appropriate exercise program, especially in terms of post-injury or post-surgery, many people are left having to guess for themselves or wading through conflicting answers that will pop up on a web search.

Imagine this: You're watching your favorite morning news show, and one day it features a trainer who explains that their new program is different than all the rest. There are new exercises you've never seen before and variations on some old favorites. The instructor or trainer is in great shape and smiles as they encourage you to "dig deep and push harder." Fast forward to six months later, and there has been no pain and your results are better than ever.

Finally, after the achy mornings, years of doctor visits, many mornings in physical therapy, and nights of hard work you've put into this new program, you feel terrific. You have almost forgotten that you ever had pain before … but then it happens again. You think to yourself, "There is no way this can be happening right now!" What you're feeling isn't the full-blown injury yet either. It's just a tightness, a dull reminder that the injury never really left. You slow the program down, ice the area nightly, stretch every morning, and even begin to pray more, but three months later, on a random morning, it happens again … only this time the pain is worse than you even remembered.

## EXERCISE/INJURY (E/I) CYCLE

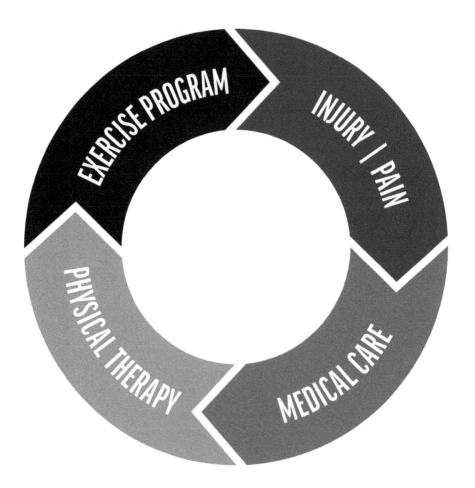

The general story above referenced one scenario that could happen along this cycle that I call the Exercise/Injury (E/I) Cycle. It is a constant hamster wheel of pain followed by relief, only to have the pain return worse or in a new, seemingly unrelated area of the body.

Many people will enter the cycle just by getting injured without ever entering an exercise program. Others will be injured while playing a sport or sustain a contact injury such as repercussions from a car accident or a hard fall. In some cases, physical therapy will be skipped over entirely, and one will go from their doctor's office right back into their same exercise or movement routines. It matters less where and how one gets on the E/I Cycle, but more about how you can get *off* of it.

## Ending the Cycle

Going back to my own story about my personal trainer and physical therapist, I've never placed blame on either the physical therapist or the personal trainer. I share my story to explain that I was stuck on the E/I Cycle with no end in sight. In my experience, most people don't even realize there is an issue or that they are stuck on this hamster wheel. Now we return to our first question of "Whose fault is this anyway?" I don't think this is your fault either, but just the fault of a fundamentally flawed system. I am also not in any way stating these fields are doing a disservice, but I *am* saying that through certain improvements, the first of which is awareness, the cycle can be broken, and the system can work better by becoming more connected and cohesive.

Currently, there is no industry mediator to bridge the gaps between all the fields on the cycle or explain the importance of detailed communication. With this understanding, you need to remove yourself from the cycle. I was able to do this for myself by studying all aspects of health, wellness, and movement and figuring out how to create a new paradigm for myself. Now, I know that you probably can't drop everything to do that for yourself. That's okay—that's why I wrote this book.

The first practical step you can take in being an agent of change in both the fitness industry and the E/I Cycle is simple *awareness*. Having an awareness of how the system works and that you're not alone in it is the first key to removing yourself from the cycle. The next key is understanding how we can improve communication in the system, what aspects you need to be aware of, what questions you need to be asking, and who you need to be talking to.

> **Having an awareness of how the system works and that you're not alone in it is the first key to removing yourself from the cycle.**

# CHAPTER 3

# Okay-ness to Wellness

*Alone, we can do so little; together, we can do so much.*
—HELEN KELLER

My third awakening happened the summer before I started graduate school. I was working for a top fitness company as a personal trainer and also working as a physical therapy aide for my mentor at the time, who I will call Dr. Thomas.

Dr. Thomas loved to quiz his aides and interns, so one day he called me into his office between appointments, and, while he was scarfing down his lunch, he asked, "What are the muscles of the rotator cuff?"

I was never good at being put on the spot, so I got nervous, my mind clouded, and I could only think of one of the four. "Supraspinatus and, ah …" I mumbled nervously.

He smiled and said, "You're working at a top club now, you have clients who pay you a lot of money, you have a degree, but you don't know all the body muscles? When you go home, look it up and get back to me tomorrow with the answer."

Dr. Thomas then leaned over to his stack of books and said, "I also want you to study this book here." He handed me a book called *How to Eat, Move, and Be Healthy!* by Paul Chek.[17] He continued by explaining, "It talks about a lot more than just a different way to exercise."

Chek's book is about all things health and wellness, yet I was amazed that the topic of exercise was only one section of the book toward the back. Instead, the majority of the book covered topics like food quality, hydration, sleep, gut health, and other forms of movement. I was hooked from the first page as my list of questions for the healthcare community continued to grow. Most exercise-related books I had encountered up to that point were dry and only meant for the exercise professional or they were only focused on aesthetics through gaining muscle or improving athletic performance through fitness training programs.[18]

In the book *Periodization Training for Sports*, a go-to in the world of sports training, the authors demonstrate how to improve performance based on phases of training. They discuss anatomical adaptation, hypertrophy, maximum strength, conversion to specific strength, maintenance, and tapering. Now, this is a great source of information if you're looking to aid your physical and athletic performance through improvements in your sports training process, but it is not as applicable for the average individual looking to improve their fitness journey. Chek's book, however, was about taking a comprehensive,

---

17     Paul Chek, *How to Eat, Move and Be Healthy!: Your Personalized 4-step Guide to Looking and Feeling Great From the Inside Out*, 1st ed. (Carlsbad, CA: C. H. E. K. Institute, 2004).

18     Tudor Bompa and Carlo Buzzichelli, *Periodization Training for Sports*, 3rd ed. (Champaign, IL: Human Kinetics, 2015).

more holistic look at wellness to create a healthy lifestyle for anyone. While much of the information in the book can be debated today, it was the concept of looking beyond exercise and basic nutrition that really opened my eyes.

After that, I began to look into everything related to Paul Chek, which took me to the biggest game-changer of them all, *The Meeting of the Minds*. This was a DVD recording of an event put on by a company called PTontheNet, where many of the top agents of change in the fitness industry had come together to speak on the new changes in the fitness and healthcare industry. Other than Paul Chek, I had not heard of any of the other featured speakers at the time, such as Tom Myers, Charles Poliquin, and Chuck Wolf.

It was here that I learned about the new findings in areas like total body wellness, holistic nutrition, the fascial system, and what would become my own niche, prehabilitation. From that day on, my world was forever changed. I would show that DVD to anybody who would watch it. It wasn't precisely what each speaker was saying that was amazing—it was how much I realized I had yet to learn. And more than that, it was how much research was out there that wasn't being discussed by anybody I knew in the fitness industry. And even more than that, it was fascinating how fitness and nutrition professionals were discussing healthcare topics because they felt there was a broken system.

## Root Causes

The root causes for America's deplorable health statistics would be too simple to place on just one area of healthcare. For example, one such consideration is in regard to healthcare quality, especially regarding hospitals. According to research from the American College of Healthcare Executives, several issues that affected quality included finances, patient safety, patient satisfaction, access to care, and doctor-related issues.[19] We must also consider quality in outpatient fields, including physical therapy and chiropractic, in addition to personal training.

Now, I've already addressed two issues that I believe play a role: the lack of communication between healthcare professionals and those in the fitness industry, but also the fact that insurance can drive medical decisions more than what is best for the individual. But from my point of view, a couple of other factors directly related to the healthcare industry that I believe need to be examined and addressed are (1) overspecialization and (2) lack of collaboration among functional experts.

## OVERSPECIALIZATION

As a society, we have created a healthcare system of specialists because, let's be honest here, no one can know everything about everything. Examples of this are seen in every field, such as how orthopedics specialize in the musculoskeletal system, neurologists specialize in the nervous system, and physical therapists specialize in musculoskeletal rehabilitation. In the allied health professions, it is the same: fitness professionals specialize in movement, aesthetics, or performance enhancement, psychologists deal with mental/emotional wellbeing, and even nutritionists and RDs specialize in dietary influences on the body. But the specialization does not stop there.

Every specialty can have its own subspecialties, such as how orthopedics has specific joint specialists and fitness has specialists

---

19   "Top Issues Confronting Hospitals," American College of Healthcare Executives, accessed September 20, 2021, https://www.ache.org/learning-center/research/about-the-field/top-issues-confronting-hospitals/top-issues-confronting-hospitals-in-2019.

who primarily focus on professional athletics or geriatric fitness, and so on. There are famous nutritionists who break away from the norm to develop plant-based-only diets, and even psychologists will argue whether it's better to practice clinical or practical psychology. This creates a model where the specialist is fine-tuned to solve any health problems that apply to their specific scope. The positive is that this type of model is necessary in a world where new research develops so quickly that there is too much information for any professional to stay up-to-date with *all* the latest findings. This model also creates a place for a person to go when they have a particular health problem that requires a deeper level of knowledge and care. The issue is that with any great progression comes the inevitable problems it begets (i.e., the unintended consequences).

The first big problem is the Law of the Instrument. "If all you have is a hammer, everything looks like a nail," said world-renowned psychologist Abraham Maslow in his seminal work *The Psychology of Science.*[20] The human body and mind are more complex than our research may ever be able to uncover. To attribute a problem, pain, or disease to only a single area of a person may cause a major misdiagnosis in the person as a whole, which is why a holistic approach makes more sense.

> To attribute a problem, pain, or disease to only a single area of a person may cause a major misdiagnosis in the person as a whole.

For example, if the pain in your left shoulder turns out to be a symptom of a tear in your labrum and it can be fixed by surgery by a highly recommended orthopedic doctor specializing in shoulder

---

20    Abraham Maslow, *The Psychology of Science: A Reconnaissance*, 1st ed. (New York: Harper Collins, 1966).

pain, that's all well and good. But *how* you got the tear, what your life becomes as a result of the tear, and what you need to do after the tear, are all questions *another* specialist would still need to address for your treatment to be complete.

As the Exercise/Injury Cycle shows, the next professional to see would most likely be a physical therapist. Their role is to cover acute rehabilitation both pre- and post-surgery (if performed). The therapist will provide strategies that work toward getting your shoulder back to its proper range of motion and make sure the shoulder is fully restored. The physical therapist treatment may include things like active and/or passive stretching, myofascial release techniques, resistance training, and/or joint mobilization/stabilization. Ideally, the exact purpose of these recommendations and what the goal of each one is for you will be explained so that you can approach them with a greater sense of ownership and purpose.

However, what else may have caused the tear, what your life is like as a result of the tear, and what to do—and not to do—in an exercise program six months after completing physical therapy, generally will not be covered by the PT or the orthopedic surgeon. In this scenario, neither professional is looking at the person *as a whole* to see where the tear is coming from or whether it is exacerbated by a poor exercise program, overuse as a result of one's job or home life, a simple movement dysfunction stemming from somewhere else in the body, a lack of nutrients in one's diet, or even if there was a better treatment protocol than surgery in the first place. Sometimes surgery could have been avoided but ends up as the go-to solution proposed as part of our "quick-fix" culture. Missing any of these factors could leave the person vulnerable to a similar or more extreme injury in the future.

## INCOMMUNICADO (LACK OF COMMUNICATION)

This leads into the second and most important problem that I've already hinted at, which is a lack of communication across all fields. The human body is far more complex than a building, and yet think about all the people involved in construction of a building: the architect, the general contractor, the electricians, the plumbers, the masons, the carpenters, and so on. If you're working on the building and all you have is a hammer, then you're going to need someone else's tools and expertise when it comes time to put in the electrical wiring. In other words, you need a full tool belt—and a team.

Likewise, having a professional network of other specialists who all assess that same person will see the problem through different professional lenses and based on their available tools. By communicating and working together, they can allow the patient to have a diagnosis from an entire toolbox full of instruments and ensure that no problem goes missing or untreated. Thus, you would not only be helping to solve the current problem at hand, but also stopping future health complications before they have a chance to develop.

Having subsections can again be very helpful, as it allows one to become a specialist and focus all of their energy into mastering one topic. You wouldn't see your general practitioner (GP) for cancer treatment; you would see your oncologist because they have spent their whole life after premed steering their learning toward how to save the lives of cancer patients. In contrast, the GP has learned a variety of different topics, and you should go see them when you have illness or symptoms of illness so that they can diagnose you and direct you toward a specialist.

The key here is the word "direct." It is uncommon practice for an orthopedic doctor to speak to your physical therapist about you and your pain in length. They write the script, and the PT takes care of the rest. The PT releases you, and you see your fitness professional, who reassesses you and takes it from there. But where is the collaboration or communication? The orthopedist learned things about you that your PT wouldn't even assess for, and your PT learned even more about your movement, which the FP would never assess or evaluate.

This also works in reverse. If you get injured while using a personal trainer or FP, that FP has known you for weeks, months, or even years. If it were common practice for the FP to speak to an orthopedic doctor about their client's exercise history, movement ability, nutritional habits, even the client's lifestyle, the orthopedist would have a much more well-rounded picture of who the patient is before they even stepped in the door. This would make the visit to the orthopedist quicker, easier, more efficient, and create a greater chance of proper and detailed diagnosis.

# The Bottom Line

The solution is having multifaceted communities of practice. Wellness already has models for this when it comes to preventative healthcare. For example, there are wellness centers you can join that employ top exercise physiologists (EPs), registered dietitians, nurse practitioners, MDs or DOs, and more. A lot of times, these centers are seen as more yoga and vegan-based "*safe spaces*," but in actuality, there is a wide range for what makes a wellness center. There are the yoga/Pilates/meditation-type facilities, but there are also centers that do screening for proper movement, take bloodwork to check vitamin and hormone levels, and put together an intuitive nutrition program for your specific needs. Both types of wellness centers share the same goals: to help you while you are still healthy and help you navigate any negative aspects of your lifestyle *before* you need a classical physician or fall ill.

However, the methods, level of professionals, and client/patient outcomes are drastically different depending on which type of facility you join. Therefore, it's imperative that you understand what you are looking for before becoming a member or purchasing a package at either of these types of wellness centers.

We'll talk more about prevention-based healthcare in Part 3, but for now, I want to focus on the critical importance of establishing proper communication channels in either one or both of these spaces. For example, packages should not have titles like you would see in a gym or nutrition practice alone, such as "Meet with our _____ professional three days a week for $500/month or two days a week for $300." They should be all-inclusive and assessment based. After all, how could you possibly know who you need to see, let alone how often you should see them until you know what exactly you need?

So let's talk about expectations for joining a wellness center. Upon arrival, you should receive an assessment by one of the medical professionals on staff. This medical professional should be well-versed in the intricacies of each service, program, and professional at the site.

Then, based on your needs and goals and their knowledge of the center, they should present you with different options. These should be titled things like "Move Better and Feel Better," "Learn a New Approach to Nutrition," and "Regeneration for the New Generation." Package titles like these would promote all-encompassing programs. They are not random packages assigned to anybody and everybody who walks into the center.

For example, "Move Better and Feel Better" may consist of different options based on different price points, but the different options would have you meet with a variety of different health/allied health and fitness professionals. It may indicate that you see the fitness professional three days a week, the registered dietitian two days a month, and have your blood drawn and analyzed by the MD before even beginning the program.

There would then be a meeting between the MD, RD, FP, and the original medical practitioner who gave your assessment and any other appropriate professional on staff who can provide proper insight. In this meeting, they would create specific action steps for what each one of them would be targeting and how the program would progress as the weeks continue and how those action steps work together. These types of meetings may happen on a weekly or monthly basis to make sure that your program is continuously tailored to your changing needs and program results. Emails and virtual calls could be made biweekly, if not more often, to keep everyone updated on your outcomes, and a shareable virtual chart would be filled out by each professional after every visit to assure you receive the most up-to-date, accurate help. And yes, forms would need to be signed, and HIPAA-compliant charts would have to be part of the programming process.

Then comes the hard part: shifting the mentality from the current overspecialized, non-holistic healthcare model to the preventative wellness holistic world. This is a topic for a whole different book because it's simply not enough to say we can just have doctors see patients more often for checkups, start wellness centers in each hospital, or have insurance pay for fitness professionals and other preventative allied health services. I'm not that much of an idealist to think it's *that* easy of a solution. Each of those ideas has multiple layers of complexity that would need to be weeded through by the entire healthcare community, and sadly, the world is not quite there yet.

The good news is the beginning of positive change is on the horizon, and sooner than later, this type of preventative healthcare model will be the new standard. The important takeaway for you is that you understand that while we are not quite at this new standard yet, you now have more information you can take into your next visit to any healthcare or allied healthcare professional to know what to expect—and what to demand from them.

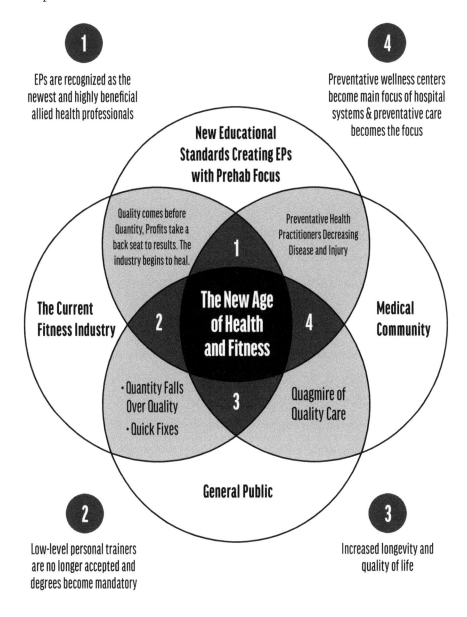

In the Allied Healthcare Overlap Diagram, you can see how all areas of healthcare and preventative wellness currently overlap with fitness. Many companies fall into the circles encompassing one or two of the major areas in healthcare and wellness, but the number gets smaller as we move more toward the middle. Very few companies overlap areas where they can then provide the multifaceted help that the world needs today.

The fitness industry is a $30 billion industry[21] that sells itself on quick fixes, especially for weight loss and aesthetics. That's a massive gross revenue being made by promoting very narrow concepts. But the important part to notice is how strongly the fitness business directly dictates the behavior of the general public yet has very little interaction with the medical community or even their own fitness educators and leaders, for that matter. This is the most obvious reason why the fitness industry still looks very similar to how it looked in the 1960s and 1970s. Despite exercise machines changing over the years[22] and new research and science, workouts today are very comparable to workouts (particularly popular bodybuilders) from the 1970s, including ones popularized by Arnold Schwarzenegger.[23] These fitness programs are not necessarily wrong to perform, but they may not be the best type of programming for the modern health and fitness professional, much less the clients they serve.

Education is always a major driver for change. If an industry discredits or ignores their educators and areas of new research that don't support their most popular, revenue-generating products and services,

---

21   Midgley, "The Six Reasons."

22   Jason Scott, "The Evolution of Fitness Equipment," Athletic Business, March 2017, https://www.athleticbusiness.com/fitness-training/the-evolution-of-fitness-equipment.html.

23   Arnold Schwarzenegger, *Encyclopedia of Modern Bodybuilding* (New York: Simon & Schuster, 1987).

then there is no room for change. The powers that be only allow the messaging to reach the general public that they find helpful for the bottom line, and their money is only funding research and projects that they can then use to sell more of their type of products. The irony here, though, is that a more holistic approach based on new research and improved communication between professionals could actually benefit the bottom line by driving exercise innovation, creation of new services, and longer retention of more dedicated and loyal clients. But these hypotheticals, even when supported by evidence, are often pushed aside when compared to what is already generating predictable revenue. And frankly, it's cheaper, easier, and "less risky" for businesses to recycle "bottom of the barrel" programs than creating something new, all of which leads to very slow change.

However, even slow change is still change. Thus, the rise of new solopreneur fitness professionals has emerged, such as prehabilitation or corrective exercise, post-orthopedic rehabilitation, cardiac rehabilitation and post-rehabilitation, functional fitness, and others. But these fields are still eclipsed by the popular domains of weight loss, aesthetics, and athletic performance, none of which help the general public as much as these other emerging domains. This is why all four large circles need to merge into almost every new project, research, and specialist/professional that overlaps with health and fitness. To return to the earlier analogy of building a building, every person involved in the process, from drawing the blueprint to painting the walls, needs to be in communication and on the same page to make the best possible building. I believe we will see stronger bodies and businesses when we can all get on the same page and use our specializations in unison.

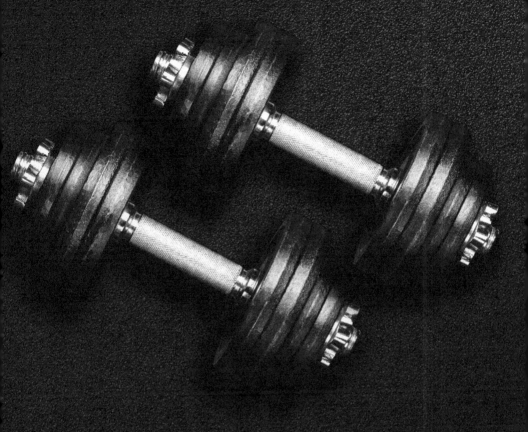

PART 2

# You Got Sold a Placebo

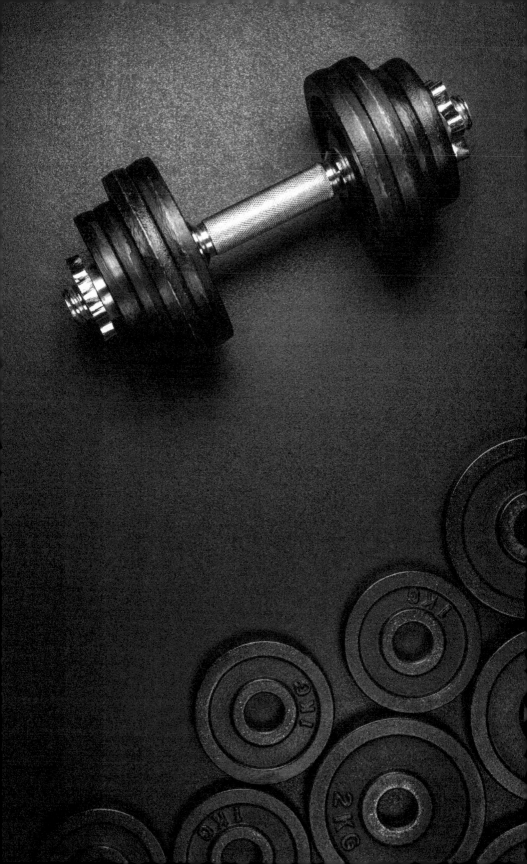

## CHAPTER 4

# Breaking Quick-Fix Mentality

*Tell me, and I forget; teach me, and I may*
*remember; involve me, and I learn.*
—BENJAMIN FRANKLIN

When I left my first corporate personal training job to open my own studio, I tried to emulate the classic personal trainer stereotype to a T. You know, the good-looking exercise fanatic with a statuesque physique who would never even think to touch a cupcake. That's what people expected, so I figured that's exactly what I should give them, proving that I was part of the problem.

How was I part of the problem? Because I knew by then that what I really wanted to do was leave the traditional fitness industry behind and do prehabilitation (prehab) with my clients, meaning that I would focus on fitness goals that could help prevent injury. But at the same time, I had a business to build and felt like I needed to "sell" myself to get people in the door, using the message of aesthetics just like everyone else was doing. So I purposefully named my business "Aesthetics to Athletics," knowing that would attract people but also knowing this was just to appease the demand of fitness culture. Honestly, I also liked that it kind of rhymed.

I knew this was the wrong message to send since, ultimately, I wanted to market the idea of prehabilitation and longevity-based fitness, but I still couldn't rid myself of the notion that people will only want to train with a fitness model and health "guru." And I wasn't completely wrong. People came in asking me how to get a six-pack, how to lose forty pounds in three months, and so on. Everyone wanted a quick fix, whereas prehab fitness is a slower, more comprehensive process. Less than a year later, I would change the name of my company to FICX Fitness, as I realized that I was only feeding into the cultural assumption that fitness equals weight loss.

As embarrassed as I am to admit it now, I remember the instances I told what I considered to be "little white lies" about my own diet, sleep, and exercise habits. I gave in to giving the "popular" advice of the time, things like "eat low carb and high protein only" or "you have to work out five days a week." I figured these were the necessary compromises I had to make in order to get my clients to trust me and gradually convert them to a prehab and holistic view of their health. It took a few more years of personal and professional development to realize what a disservice I was doing to my clients.

By telling them the "white lies" that I *never* ate dessert, that I *always* got eight to nine hours of sleep, and that I *never* trained in a bodybuilding style, I was limiting their beliefs as to what they could achieve for themselves. Instead of presenting them with other options more specific to their needs, their age, their lifestyle, and their goals, I was letting them believe the only road to health was by following a strict and ascetic lifestyle.

Side by side with this view of strict fitness and nutrition are the conventional programs advertised by popular trainers. These are the ones you see all over the media that start with high-intensity movements which, within the first thirty minutes, leave you with only two options: pass out or throw up. While their intentions may be good, this style of fitness limits the potential impact an authentic fitness coach can have on their clients. Their influence can—and should—extend well outside of just the weight room. A better physique and weight loss represent only a small part of what engaging in a health and fitness program should be. But in the beginning, I felt like I had to "go with the flow" if my clients were going to respect me.

> A better physique and weight loss represent only a small part of what engaging in a health and fitness program should be.

I learned later on that it was actually freeing for my clients to know that I was human too, that I had a lot of the same struggles as them. Once I began to open up about this, my clients actually appreciated me more for being real with them. It allowed them to realize that a healthy lifestyle is achievable when you *do* have a cupcake or two, or when you skip a couple of days at the gym, or if you want to do some bicep curls for aesthetics, even if your main goal is to move better and feel better.

I had to evolve in how I coached my clients, and the evolution of a new age in the fitness industry will give rise to the next generation of fitness coaching that moves us away from a culture of "quick fixes." After all, it would be foolish to think that our culture of fast food, HIIT classes, and sedentary jobs are going to become a thing of the past any time soon, so we need to explore the main factors in fitness that will help push us in a much better direction, starting with what you need to know *today* to start taking positive action and some control back in your life.

# Coming Together

In the last two chapters, we discussed how all healthcare and allied healthcare industries continually focus on improving their current treatment methods, including how each specialist does a phenomenal job at helping patients with conditions their specialty can treat. Now let's explore how much better the results could be if each specialty communicated with one another.

As we discussed earlier, doctors rarely speak to the physical therapists about each patient they refer. Consequently, all that the physical therapist has to work with at the beginning of treatment is the basic information the doctor wrote down concerning the diagnosis and any test results. But there is always a lot more to a person than what can be written down briefly on a prescription, leaving the PT with no other option than to run specific assessments to determine their treatment protocol based on an incomplete view of the patient. Keep in mind that the body is one interconnected unit: the psychological, physical, and even spiritual self are all one. But unless they have all the information about a patient, it easily creates a situation where the physical therapist could be treating symptoms but not getting to the root cause of the problem.

After physical therapy, unless you're in the rare situation where the PT has exercise professionals in their network, you are left to figure out the best way to get back to being fit on your own. Even in that rare case, the physical therapist rarely ever calls the exercise professional to discuss your injury rehabilitation or the current status of any risk you might have for further injury. This type of direct communication is even less common than the MD/PT communicating with one another. So although most of your life will be spent *outside* of the medical professional's care, none of the professionals ever discuss your physical status with the professionals who will see you more often—the fitness professional—to help guide you down the road to your future self. Moreover, it is essential to remember that the average fitness professional does not currently engage in a complete assessment or movement screenings that aid in creating a holistic view of your needs.

Moral of the story: without medical guidance or direction, the fitness professional could lead you down a path that will land you right back in that doctor's office very quickly. And if it does, you would want your FP communicating with that doctor since that FP knows a lot more about your day-to-day habits and progress than a doctor will ever know through sporadic, annual visits and quick examinations. When all the health and fitness professionals come together, it will create a better result for them and create a much better outcome for you.

# Fitness Professionals on the Frontline

The next generation of fitness coaching takes the idea of a personal trainer to a level never thought to be possible, one that I think can rival or surpass all other allied health professionals. Instead of giving in to—and exploiting—a culture of quick fixes that actually promotes the communication breakdown between professionals, FPs can fill in the gap and lead the way to a fitness culture that looks at a client's long-term health journey, one where "quick fixes" are no longer necessary.

The way I see it, fitness professionals should take their place on the frontline of defense against a client's unhealthy lifestyle and be their first ally in the quest for longevity and quality of life. Think about it this way: among all of the allied health professionals we've mentioned—PTs, chiros, specialists—you see your FP the most often. Your time together might range from one to four sessions a week for as short as a few months to as long as consistent training for decades. Also, unlike the other allied fields that you see sporadically or only when seeking treatment, you see your FP regardless of your current health situation or life stage. Beyond that, the reason the FP can be so "omnipresent" is that, even within the fitness industry, there can be FPs with different specializations, ranging from prehabilitation to general fitness to post-rehabilitation. The specific type of fitness professional you see will vary depending on your life stage, injury stage, and specialty you may need.

Thankfully, the specialization model is changing so that one general FP/EP can be equipped to effectively treat people at all stages of life. This idea ties the different disciplines together and helps solve the problem of miscommunication between professionals while raising the bar on what the standard fitness professional embodies. Moreover, the true potential of the field is still far from optimal since only the popular specializations of aesthetics and athletics are currently well-researched while the rest of the field remains largely under-researched.

Until this model evolves further, wherein the field can assess and treat people well *before* they have any injury or disease, we are not fulfilling its potential to contribute to the amelioration of America's dreadful health statistics. This is especially true in regards to obesity and the medical conditions that are specifically linked to it, such as high blood pressure, sleep apnea, and diabetes. According to the data from the National Health and Nutrition Examination Survey in

2017–2018, the age-adjusted prevalence of obesity in adults was 42.4 percent and severe obesity in adults was 9.2 percent.[24]

Remember, a health and fitness professional's greatest weapon on the frontline of health is that they can also cover a wide range of other health-related subjects with their clients, therefore, the multidisciplinary approach to health and wellness should be prioritized, especially in today's fast-paced society.[25] The topics they could address might include everything from essential nutrition, habit change, sleep patterns, and stress management—all factors that play a significant role in the development of disease[26] and muscular degeneration. In addition to the benefits seen from a detailed exercise prescription, covering these topics preventatively will allow clients to significantly lower their risk for injury or disease before there is even a reason for concern.

## Being Proactive Instead of Reactive

Another issue related to our "quick-fix" culture is that we tend to be reactive to a problem, only responding to it once it arises rather than being proactive to prevent the problem from arising. It's the mentality of "Why worry about something when there's nothing to worry about?" when we should be thinking, "How can I reduce my worries by making sure I won't have more to worry about?"

In the end, the goal in the new age of fitness is for FPs to lead their

24  Craig M. Hales, Margaret D. Carroll, Cheryl D. Fryar, and Cynthia L. Ogden , *Prevalence of Obesity and Severe Obesity Among Adults: United States, 2017–2018*, NCHS Data Brief No. 360, February 2020.

25  Pedram Shojai, *The Urban Monk: Eastern Wisdom and Modern Hacks to Stop Time and Find Success, Happiness, and Peace* (New York: Rodale Books, 2016).

26  Camila Hirotsu, Sergio Tufik, and Monica Levy Andersen, "Interactions between Sleep, Stress, and Metabolism: From Physiological to Pathological Conditions," *Sleep Science* 8, no. 3 (November 2015): 143–152, https://doi.org/10.1016/j.slsci.2015.09.002.

clients directly into the holy grail of a preventative health mindset: becoming proactive rather than reactive. Instead of "I need to go to the gym because I'm thirty pounds overweight," it should be, "I need to go to the gym so I don't become overweight."

Where this gets tricky, though, is being able to prove scientifically that the proactive approach works. After all, how do you show results for a disease or injury that has been prevented? It's easy to sell somebody a pain reliever after they have a headache, but they're much harder to sell when you tell somebody they are "at risk" for headaches. Generally, people don't want to do anything until they see the problem, so while you can show research on the effectiveness of a pain reliever on people dealing with a headache, it's much more difficult to show how proper diet, exercise, and sleep prevented the headache from happening in the first place.

Instead, we should be thinking of it the same way we think of car maintenance. It takes time and financial investment to get your oil changed in your car, getting the tune-up done, putting on new tires in a timely fashion. But you do those things (hopefully) because it prevents a bigger, more expensive problem from occurring. In the long run, changing your oil regularly is a lot cheaper and convenient than replacing an engine, and getting new tires in a timely fashion will help prevent a possible blowout that could cause an accident—or leave you stranded.

Fitness is similar, then, where the evidence is currently more anecdotal rather than scientific or provable. People can attest to feeling better, having more energy, sleeping better, seeing their blood pressure improve, and so on as a result of making healthier lifestyle choices. But to help convince other professionals and the public to move from reactive to proactive, the industry will have to move beyond anecdotal evidence to data-based evidence. As things stand now, we can't *prove* that we prevented someone from tearing their ACL or prevented cardiac arrest.

I think that the best possible answer to this conundrum is utilizing proper assessments and then following up with regular reassessments. In this way, it is possible to actually track the risk reduction ensuing from the FP's plan for the client. Thankfully, new advances in the health and fitness fields have already created evaluations that show risk for injury and pain. Such evaluations in combination with other health testing performed at the original assessment stage can aid in showing reduced health risks throughout the exercise program and arm the fitness professional with another tool that sets them apart from their distant cousin, the personal trainer. Therefore, when data gathered from an FP can be compared to existing data of health problems experienced by those who are not working with an FP, we will be able to show proof of prevention. In that way, it would be like comparing tooth decay in people who only brush their teeth to those who brush their teeth, floss, and go for semiannual dentist checkups.

Granted, it will likely take a couple more generations of the fitness industry for us to develop the full range of tools and data objectives needed between FPs and the medical and allied medical communities to back up this preventative approach. In some ways, I suppose that science has to catch up to some of these changes that are being implemented in the industry, but that's not really a bad thing, the way I see it. For now, I believe FPs must make incremental change by working with one person at a time to create a mind shift from building abs to building healthier lives.

# Relational Bonding

On that note, another tool that is exclusive to the FP is the amount of time they can spend one-on-one with their clients and the quality of bonding that can develop. An average of 1–4 training session days per week over the course of a year could equal 130 days spent training together. Sharing almost one-third of your year with somebody allows for them to truly get to know one another on a deeper level than what a doctor or specialist is able to do.

This amount of time allows the FP and client to build a full 360-degree view of each other as whole people, which should encourage trust within the pursuit of holistic health. This allows the FP in particular to be able to track their client's progress, mental health, and even social health that would be nearly impossible for the client's doctor to know—unless they happen to be best friends with their doctor, I guess. The doctor may only see a client once a year for an annual checkup or when they're sick, the PT may only see them when they're injured, but the FP has the special opportunity to see the client regularly and develop an atmosphere of transparency and openness. That's not something I think any FP should take lightly!

The way I see it, the most effective fitness professionals should be able to tell you about their client's whole lives. They may know their client's relationship with their spouse, their favorite vacations, preferred restaurants, sleep habits, worst memories, or even their "guilty pleasures" like favorite treats or music. This is highlighted as one of the four cornerstones of Co-Active Coaching: focus on the whole person.[27]

---

27   Ann Betz, "Co-Active Coaching and the Brain: Neuroscience Research Supports the Efficacy of the Co-Active Model," Coactive.com, August 1, 2012, https://www.beaboveleadership.com/wp-content/uploads/2012/11/Co-Active-Coaching-and-The-Brain-final.pdf.

A Co-Active Coach does not see the client simply in terms of their profession, but focuses on the entire individual and their life outside of the gym as a husband, wife, father, mother, sports enthusiast, avid cook, or whatever else inspires and motivates them as individuals.

This relationship gives the client an opportunity to vent about everything they otherwise would have to keep stuffed deep down and may help in creating a feeling of emotional release. This type of understanding allows the FP to have a more in-depth view of their client that includes discovering why a person is the way they are, how they ended up at their current state of health, what could happen to them without change, and exactly what direction to take.

It's not uncommon for a fitness professional to become close, possibly even too close, with their client, given the amount of time they spend forming a strong bond with one another, so it's essential at this point that the FP remains a true professional. Now, I know where your mind may be headed, as we've all heard the classic stereotype of personal trainers sometimes dating their clients, but please note this is *not* what the focus is here. Yes, to be a true professional, one should never date a client, and it's terrible I even have to mention it, but what I am discussing is the tendency or temptation FPs sometimes face to go *outside* of their scope of practice.

To use an extreme but clear example, you might imagine an FP notices their client coming into the gym over the course of a month appearing depressed. Maybe the client even opens up during this time about losing an important relationship, feeling sad all of the time, and so on. While it's okay for an FP to listen to their client and allow them to share, it would be inappropriate for the FP to start diagnosing the client and say, "You sound like you're struggling with depression. You should try some antidepressants."

Now, there are certain certifications that FPs can obtain that allow the discussion of essential nutrition, sleep habits, or behavior change, but there is a limit to what an FP can offer advice on, and these parameters may differ state to state. For example, discussing the nutrition habits of somebody with a health issue such as diabetes or someone who is on multiple medications is always best left to a registered dietitian. Likewise, listening to a client and learning about their personal life is often a part of the day-to-day, but giving psychological advice or relationship advice falls out of our scope of practice. I say all this because even though there will be one standard of fitness professional, the FP must remain within their scope of practice.[28]

For example, a registered dietitian can recommend certain exercises, but it's outside of their scope to do the actual training on those exercises. Likewise, FPs can recommend the government guidelines to a healthy diet or some general nutrition advice, but they should steer clear of developing detailed nutritional plans for clients. Not to sound redundant, but this is yet another reason why a network of allied medical and medical professionals is so integral and that the communication between them should be robust so that the FP can lead their client down a path of success, even if that means referring them to another professional. To be precise, it is the future fitness professional who takes a proactive approach to communication because they will remain the only profession to have so much interaction with their clients while they are still healthy.

This begs the question: With all the potential influence a fitness professional can have, why isn't this standard practice in every gym or exercise program? The answer to this question isn't as simple as blaming the fitness business, DVD/online program companies, fitness certification boards, or the trainers themselves. Remember, it's a com-

---

28  Justin Kompf, Nick Tumminello, and Spencer Nadolsky, "Scope of Practice for Personal Trainers," *Personal Trainer Quarterly* (PTQ) 1, no. 4: 4–8, https://www.researchgate.net/publication/288327851_The_scope_of_practice_for_the_personal_trainer.

bination of each group being partially at fault, mixed with the fact that there is currently no standard governing body to set guidelines of who is qualified to enter the fitness field and the underlying culture of quick fixes and quick profits.

In the next chapter, we will delve more into what created the fitness industry's current standards and the main areas that need to be addressed to cause an immediate change. The critical takeaway here is to see how the allied health field of fitness, which has so much potential to help, has turned into a profit-over-people model. This has created a flawed system that has bastardized the role of an authentic fitness professional, compromising many trainers who have entered the field for the wrong reasons and may not be properly qualified.

# The Rise of the Quick Fix

I'm not a huge television person myself, but my favorite thing to watch on TV is infomercials. I know that sounds a little unusual, but I specifically enjoy fitness infomercials, not because they are informational, but because I see them as comedy. Some have told me I'm too harsh when it comes to evaluating fitness products, but I just can't stand products created to manipulate the consumer. It takes the newly motivated person who really wants to be healthier and drains them of their excitement, time, and money, only so the quick-fix company can profit.

My "favorite" example is the late-night hour-long infomercials that push the idea that people don't have time to exercise. Maybe you've seen it before. A sweaty guy or girl pops up on your screen with three or four grinning lackeys in the background. The primary instructor has a headset on and, from the very start, has extra-high energy. Maybe you're sitting on your couch in sweats, trying to relax after a hard day, and they scream words at you like, "Get up, let's go!" and "Everybody can do this from the comfort of their own home!"

First of all, you are nice and comfortable, relaxing in your own home, but it's only *now* that you feel *un*comfortable. These ads shame you into feeling like you're doing something wrong or not enough. But that isn't even the worst part, because next they say, "You don't need an hour at the gym to work out. Give us ten minutes a day!" They're implying that by doing their high-intensity workout for ten minutes a day, you'll look like them.

They don't disclose anything about their personal exercise program that they are doing *behind* the cameras for hours each day so that they can look at that. I mean, think about it … do you really think *they* are only exercising for ten minutes a day?

But to make sure they sell you, they aim to *relate* to you, saying things like, "We know you're too busy to work out for longer than ten minutes, so we made this just for you!" So by now, you've been shamed and lied to, but to top it off, they patronize you. You're sitting on the couch watching this for over twenty minutes. Another thing to think about: the company bought an hour-long slot on late-night TV, so they *know* you actually have longer than ten minutes to work out, or else they would have just bought a ten-minute slot, right? This is the marketing ploy that is so ubiquitous when you play the game of the "quick-fix" fitness routine.

Everything from thirty-day summer body DVDs to thirty-second abs videos also creates an internal competition that has become the fitness industry's underlying goal. Programs seem to be promising faster and faster results because there is an assumption in "quick-fix" culture that the quicker the results, the better the program, right? They know many people will answer *yes* to this question, which is why the fitness industry continues to use these methods.

Sure, there are positives to an accelerated program. These might include being more cost-effective, the opportunity to participate without any direct professional instruction, ability to begin without any assessment, or the possibility they can get you to your aesthetic results faster, *assuming* you can make it through the program without being hurt. Ironically, price notwithstanding, those very same factors that make the programs fast are often what makes them not only ineffective but even counterproductive in the long run. But the truth is that many factors are involved in creating a quality exercise program and a quicker time to the desired results is only *one* to consider—and nowhere near the most important factor.

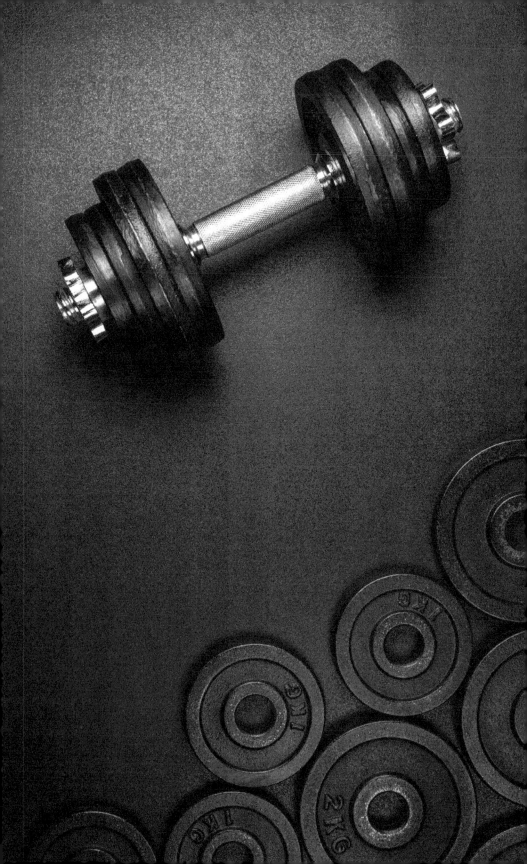

# CHAPTER 5

# Quality Over Quantity

*Be a yardstick of quality. Some people aren't used to*
*an environment where excellence is expected.*
—STEVE JOBS

When I launched my first company back in 2014, it was a fitness studio where I wanted to show that I covered all aspects of fitness. My first location was in Long Island, New York, way in the back of a wellness facility located on top of a shopping center. The wellness center had complimentary services that ranged from yoga and nutrition to meditation and reiki. I purposely chose to sublet from this location because I thought if I were inside a wellness center, the clients who would come to see me would already have a more holistic view of fitness.

One of the first clients to walk through my door was a woman named Alexandra, Alex for short. She was a 5'5", 140-pound, forty-five-year-old woman with a husband who worked in New York City.

Alex was a yoga student at the wellness center, so naturally, when she wanted fitness advice, she was directed to me. She was a former student-athlete, an aspiring yoga instructor, and an active mother to her two sons, ages fourteen and sixteen. As she walked into my studio for her initial assessment on a hot August day, I could already see a small limp in her gait and a rounding to her shoulders. Before getting into the evaluation, we talked a little about her busy life on Long Island, how she felt about the wellness center, and how yoga made her feel.

"I'm always exhausted and constantly busy because I still need to pick up and drop off my kids everywhere," she expressed to me. "Yoga is my outlet. It keeps me feeling grounded and strong."

Alex continued about how even though she felt good and was overall healthy, she knew she needed other types of fitness to accomplish her goals. I was excited as we went through the preliminary forms before the assessment began because I felt she would be a great client: she was aware of her body with a knowledge base of the right outcome of fitness. And because she was recommended to me by the center, she already knew what I did in my specific niche as a corrective exercise specialist and exercise physiologist.

So once the waivers and readiness evaluations were signed, I turned the page and asked the first question with a smile on my face:

"Okay, Alex, so why don't you tell me what your goals are?"

"Well," she replied, "I need to lose five to seven pounds before a wedding I'm attending in September."

The smile from my face must have visibly disappeared, as her head slightly tilted to the side and she continued a little slower and more cautiously, "Is that possible?"

The potentially perfect client—young, active, strong, with just some muscular imbalance, and what she called "normal aches and pain"—asked me if she can lose five to seven pounds by September when it was already mid-August. We could have worked on her structural issues, improved her yoga practice, reduced her stress levels, increased her longevity, and the quality of that longevity, but instead, she heard "fitness" and thought "weight loss." Not only weight loss, but quick, purely aesthetic weight loss.

Now, don't hear me wrong, it's okay to have a weight loss goal, and many of my clients do. The issue is that weight loss should be seen as a *result*, not the primary goal. For example, if you come to me and want to lose twenty pounds over the course of six months, but I see during the assessment that you've got some movement dysfunctions, then my focus is going to be on corrective exercise techniques over the first three to six weeks so that you can move better. Once that's been addressed, not only should you feel better, but the exercise itself will make a greater impact and will help lead to the desired weight loss.

I believe quick-fix and weight-loss-focused programs will gradually become a thing of the past and have earned their place in the dustbin of history. Why do I say that? Well, you can see how the "quick-fix" mindset engulfed Alex, and upon further analysis of her goals, she did eventually change her mind about only focusing on weight loss. And it really came down to how she was influenced by the Quality over Quantity Principle (QOQ).

# Quality over Quantity, not Quantity over Quality

To truly understand the QOQ principle, you first need to understand the difference in symmetrical and asymmetrical exercises. Symmetrical exercises are those in which both sides of your body do exactly the same movement, such as bench press and back squats. Asymmetrical exercises then are those where the two sides of your body are doing different movements, such as lifting a dumbbell on one side only, where the movement can create some imbalance. For example, you can saw unilaterally for a one-sided exercise or saw bilaterally for a more symmetrical exercise.

As I mentioned earlier, I always want to help clients learn to move better, which is why I like to build on a foundation of asymmetrical structures to better identify problems in someone's movements. These are the type of movements that can potentially lead to an injury and also better reflect everyday life movements, such as reaching for a glass on a high shelf or climbing in and out of your car where you're not squatting evenly but twisting, turning, and using upper body strength mostly on one side of the body to complete the motion. At its core, movement is a behavior, and a fitness program can be designed to address those imbalances since improved movement is key to long-term progress.

The QOQ principle emphasizes a direct correlation between the quality of one's exercise form and proper movement when placed under a program of continuously increasing quantity of reps and sets over time. One of the biggest current debates in fitness is the integrity of HIIT programs such as Zumba, tabata workouts, OrangeTheory, or CrossFit. Again, I believe that fitness should be about a person's specific goals and finding the proper coach to help them reach those goals safely and effectively, regardless of the program. But with that said, CrossFit does provide a perfect example of an inverse QOQ, that is, Quantity over Quality.

Just in case you've never heard of it, CrossFit is structured around specific diets like paleo, concepts like the WOD (workout of the day), and what its founder, Greg Glassman, considers functional exercises. The benefit of CrossFit to the exercise field is the aspect of community that is often missing from traditional gyms. As big corporate gyms (LA Fitness, Planet Fitness, etc.) began to rise in the 1990s, the days of strong, boutique fitness studio communities fell apart and, with them, the loss of a sense of community.

However, with CrossFit's rise and what they call boxes (gyms), these smaller, "everyone doing one workout" shops have brought back a sense of community to the world of fitness. This strengthened a model for new smaller gyms to adapt and attract new members who want more than just a place to work out. They also want that sense of belonging.

The flipside with many HIIT programs, though, is what I consider a "one-size-fits-all" approach. In CrossFit, the emphasis on paleo ignores the fact that it might not be the best diet for everybody's health goals, though I'm of the opinion that no diet is the "best" diet. By 2030, there may be some new fad diet that CrossFit adopts, which I think would still be an incorrect approach. Remember, the idea is to find a registered dietitian who can help you navigate through all the garbage flooding the nutrition field and help you find *your* right eating habits. Again, it's not that paleo is terrible—it's just not right for most people, in my experience.

The next issue is closer to my heart: the WOD. I dislike anything even remotely close to a workout of the day. The reasons run along a large spectrum, ranging from the possible cause of rhabdomyolysis[29] to the previously stated idea that people are all different and need a personally designed workout program. Now, before you think I'm just picking on CrossFit, I think this even goes for DVDs/online workout programs that change the workout daily or even weekly.

---

29  Karel Heytens, Willem D. Ridder, Jan De Bleecker, Luc Heytens, and Jonathan Baets, "Exertional Rhabdomyolysis: Relevance of Clinical and Laboratory Findings, and Clues for Investigation," *Anaesthesia and Intensive Care* 47, no. 2 (2019): 128–133, https://doi.org/10.1177/0310057X19835830.

Instead, I think you can do different exercises every day, but they should loop back and follow the same routine in the next few days or the following week for at least four and no more than eight weeks. For example, a repeating routine could look something like this:

| DAY | WORKOUT TYPE | EXERCISES |
|---|---|---|
| DAY 1 | Lower Body | Single leg deadlifts<br>Kettlebell swings<br>Goblet squats<br>Lateral lunges |
| DAY 2 | Upper Body | Weighted push-ups<br>Landmine single arm shoulder press<br>Bent-over rows<br>Plank reaches<br>TRX bicep curls and tricep press |
| DAY 3 | Full Body/Functional | Warding patterns<br>Chops and lifts<br>Half-kneeling KB halo<br>Turkish Get-up<br>Farmers walks |
| DAY 4 | Technique/Form Mastering | KB swing form<br>Squat correctives<br>Brettzel Arm Bar<br>Exercise ball single leg bridge<br>Alternate side resistance band dead bugs |
| DAY 5 | Rest Day | - |
| REPEAT | | |

Now, the chart is simply an example to give you an idea of what a workout rotation can look like, not a recommendation for *you*. I can't say it enough—whatever you do, you need to develop a workout routine with your FP that represents your specific needs and goals. But this gives you a good idea of how you can have some diversity in your exercise plan without it being so unpredictable you can't track how you're progressing. In fact, the idea is that you would repeat your schedule for at least the next four to eight weeks, and with each successive week, you would do the same movements but increase the resistance or quantity as needed, so long as you are maintaining good form.

The body takes at least four to six weeks for the neuromuscular system to adapt to a new exercise program and six to eight weeks for the muscular system to reach its full potential.[30] So if you change your workout every day for weeks on end, your body never gets a chance to maximize the results of the routine. It really doesn't even give the body a chance to catch up and learn the movement entirely. The neuromuscular system plays a more significant role in maintaining proper form than the muscular system alone. So if you

> The neuromuscular system plays a more significant role in maintaining proper form than the muscular system alone.

change your routine before the four-week mark, you are almost guaranteed to never master the form of those exercises, even if you revisit them every so often but without intentionality.

30    David A. Gabriel, Gary Kamen, and Gail Frost, "Neural Adaptations to Resistive Exercise," *Sports Med* 36 (2006): 133–149, https://doi.org/10.2165/00007256-200636020-00004; Toshio Moritani and Herbert A. deVries, "Neural Factors Versus Hypertrophy in the Time Course of Muscle Strength Gain," *American Journal of Physical Medicine and Rehabilitation* 58, no. 3 (1979): 115–130, https://paulogentil.com/pdf/Neural%20factors%20versus%20hypertrophy%20in%20the%20time%20course%20of%20muscle%20strength%20gain.pdf.

This is where I think CrossFit and other HIIT programs err on the side of thinking that the more workouts you do—or the more reps in a workout—the better it is for you, instead of focusing on doing a smaller amount of workouts but doing them really well so that you're maximizing the benefit of the exercise.

This idea crosses over into popular functional exercises, meaning exercises that are designed to train the body for activities you might do in your day-to-day life, like squatting or lifting movements as I described earlier when discussing asymmetrical movements. But like the term "holistic," the meaning of "functional workout" has been co-opted so often that the argument can be made that "functional" means *anything* you do in your daily life, from how you moved as a baby to moving with the perfect mechanics.

So it's important to note that we are referring to the way Gray Cook defines function in his video collection called *Assessing Movement: A Contrast in Approaches and Future Directions*.[31] Here, Cook defines function as "a state where we pursue physical excellence without an inappropriate side effect." He goes on to say, "If a person specializes in a particular endeavor, there's greater potential for side effects. But if that's the plan, we can manage it. It's really hard to define function, so we usually invert it and try to define *dysfunction*. We're not trying to predict function. We're trying to catch dysfunction in a bottleneck that may or may not add unnecessary risk or poor adaptability."

Because the definition of "functional" gets blurry in many HIIT programs, it lacks intentionality. There is nothing wrong with functional exercises in and of themselves, but the QOQ Principle means that they should be used in alignment with a specific goal and emphasize form.

---

31    Stuart McGill, Gray Cook, and Craig Liebenson, *Assessing Movement: A Contrast in Approaches & Future Directions*, January 25th, 2014, Stanford University, Palo Alto, California, DVD, 5:40.

When you analyze many HIIT programs in their approach to sets and reps, it becomes clearer that they are not typically following the QOQ Principle. Although not every HIIT workout is done under a clock, many are. For example, a WOD routine may say "For Time," meaning you would try to complete all the exercises in as short a time as possible. For example, The Murph is a currently popular workout that consists of a one-mile run, followed by one hundred pull-ups, two hundred push-ups, three hundred squats, and finishes with another one-mile run, all "for time." You might get tired just reading that, or you may look at it and think it sounds easy. Later on, you can look up some videos if you need to, but for now, you can just do a visualization with me.

You put on your two-year-old gym shoes that have been sitting in the closet for most of that time, and you start on the first mile run. Maybe you have a background in track, were athletic in high school, or used to run for fun, so the mile is tough but not impossible. Next up, the one hundred pull-ups. Again, let's say you've continuously exercised for years, so a hundred pull-ups are not exactly easy but doable for you.

Now, you're on to the push-ups. This is the easiest to picture in your head. Exhausted already, you get the first thirty down, 170 left to go. You muster up the energy for another fifty. Still 120 left to go. Here's where inverse QOQ (Quantity over Quality) kicks in. As you do the next fifty push-ups, you start to lose good form. Maybe your back is sinking a little lower to the ground than when you started, or your chest is lifting before your hips, or your head is tucked in and dropping to the floor, causing your spine to be out of alignment. But you push through and just do it. No pain, no gain, right?

Now it's time for three hundred squats. You've watched the how-to videos and even had a coach teach you the proper form. So the first 150 are comfortable, and you're just happy they aren't push-ups anymore. But the second half is a different story. Do you feel yourself becoming fatigued? Do you feel your back arching again? Is your head tilted back, looking up at the ceiling, trying to help you move upward? Do you even care what muscle groups you are using? Or are your knees locking out so hard you can feel the pressure in your face?

All right, we don't even need to finish the final set, let alone the last run, so you can rest now. Did you feel your form falling apart as time went on and the reps increased? That's the essence of inverse QOQ where quantity trumps quality.

So the same would go for any online workout where you see a timer begin to count down. This is why when you hear "thirty-minute workout" or "sixty-second abs," my two cents is that you should already start to question the long-term effectiveness of the program. A good plan and coach wouldn't base an entire program off time or high repetitions. Especially not a randomly generated number of reps or a random amount of time. And by random, I mean not explicitly designed for *your* body and goals from a qualified fitness professional.

## QUICK PROGRAM PROGRESSION

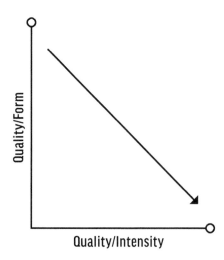

As you can see in the diagram, our culture of "quick fixes" is linked to a fitness system where quantity of reps and high intensity movement has become popular to the detriment of quality and form. So do you think it's really any surprise that we often unintentionally set ourselves up for injury when trainers should be helping us be healthier?

The big takeaway for a true QOQ Principle is that form will always matter more than repetitions. When you begin to see fitness as a lifelong journey, you'll notice how many of the most popular programs today just don't make any sense because they stress quantity instead of quality. And it's easy to think you're really accomplishing something in those programs because you probably feel exhausted at the end of them. But if the goal of fitness is consistency and longevity, then you should want your form and quality to increase over time and throughout your workouts, not decrease.

So one of the problems with focusing only on quantity or speed is that if you are exercising with progressively worse form, then you're training your neuromuscular system to use bad form, inefficient movement, and then that will project into your daily life and your functional movements. So all those push-ups you did with your head dropping down, your back getting out of alignment, could later translate to you throwing out your back when pushing yourself up off the floor while playing with your kids. Or doing deadlifts with poor form could lead to you tearing a tendon while picking up a heavy bag, putting you right back into the dreaded E/I Cycle.

> We have no problem with Quality over Quantity in other areas of life, like the workplace or family, but we stay stuck on the idea of "more is better" when it comes to fitness.

What's interesting is that we have no problem with Quality over Quantity in other areas of life, like the workplace or family, but we stay stuck on the idea of "more is better" when it comes to fitness. We celebrate completing more reps, more miles, more weight than the day before without thinking about whether it is helping us improve our health or considering whether we might be setting ourselves up for injury. But if the goal of fitness is to feel better and move better, then a mile run with good form will always be preferable to a five-mile run that ends in you limping to the doctor's office. The emphasis that "more is better" is as outdated as "no pain, no gain" when we should be moving to the belief that "better is better."

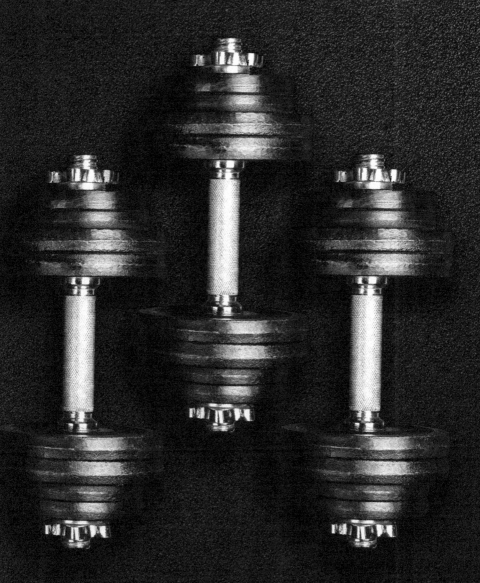

**PART 3**

# The Future of Fitness

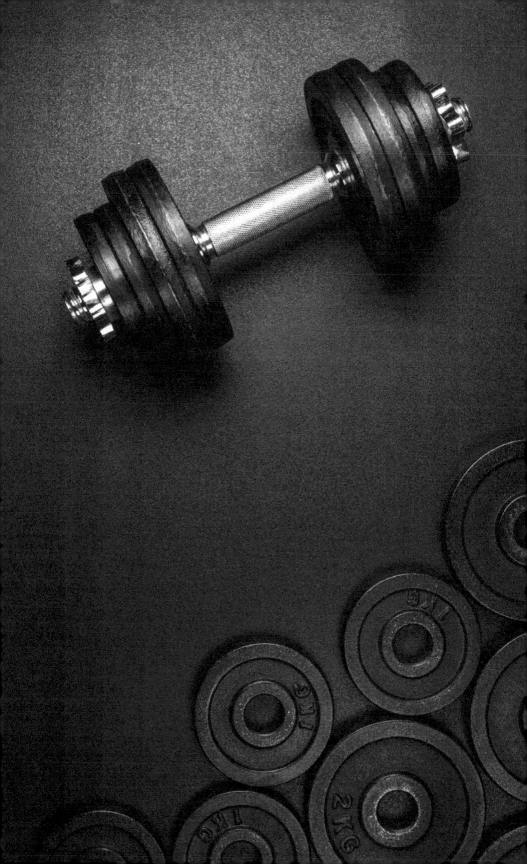

# CHAPTER 6

# Making It Feel Right

*Change happens when the pain of staying the
same is greater than the pain of change.*
—TONY ROBBINS

In 2008, the stock price for Domino's Pizza had hit an all-time low. Even though the company was investing in keeping up a positive brand image, they were losing customers. They couldn't pinpoint any changes that needed to be made with the pizza itself or with their marketing. But these were the external parts of the business, the part that the public sees. What needed to change was *inside* the company itself.

Once they realized this, they started making internal changes, implementing new technology to make the ordering process more efficient and more engaging for customers. The pizzas didn't change, but the process did. Four years later, they were profitable again because they had changed their view of their customer and how to serve them from the inside out.[32]

Now, you probably didn't pick up a fitness book expecting a story about pizza, but here it is. The way I see it, though, it's similar with the fitness industry. It's not the exercises themselves that need to change specifically, but the way that the industry is approaching the public. The way I see it, until the industry decides to change from the inside out, it will continue to fall short at almost every turn even though it is a field with the potential to create a major positive impact on the world. Meanwhile, the public is constantly bombarded with messages about the best way to enhance health from illegitimate and non-authoritative sources who have little or no expertise, like the latest Insta-famous influencer, or even worse, charlatans selling the latest snake oil solution.

The media is constantly flooded with information about how you should eat, exercise, sleep, and socialize, as they need to fill the twenty-four-hour news cycle with the latest "breaking news" or create clicks on their website that will generate ad revenue. Exercise and nutrition seem to be popular filler topics when there isn't a major national or global event to cover. So as I've mentioned before, there isn't a qualifying line for who a real fitness professional is and who isn't. Thus, when your morning show or talk show host brings on an "expert," you should approach that label with some level of skepticism. At minimum, they will probably only present their niche or product rather than a competing perspective or potential alternatives. This can make it difficult—nearly impossible—to find quality information or establish who to trust.

---

32   Profit&, "7 Real-Life Examples of Successful Change Management in Business," September 20, 2019, https://insights.profitand.com/blog/real-life-examples-of-successful-change-management-in-business.

Upon closer inspection, you may notice the newest exercise craze or the hot diet plan of the year seems to be eerily similar to their predecessors. A spin bike is a spin bike, whether you put bands on it or a computer monitor. A thirty-minute at home HIIT workout is very similar to a twenty-minute, or ten-minute workout. The thirty-day restart programs are always similar to the ninety-day programs, just capitalizing on the "quick-fix" culture to grab your attention. These examples might seem

> Upon closer inspection, you may notice the newest exercise craze or the hot diet plan of the year seems to be eerily similar to their predecessors.

obvious, but they are at the core of just about every new product you see on the market today. But we don't need new packaging around the same product—we need new, innovative products. The same goes for the entire structure of the fitness industry.

Think back to the last exercise program you looked up or saw advertised. Did it sound something like "complete X number of sets and Y number of reps in Z amount of time" or, more simply, "do this exercise for X seconds"? Did the program consist of some combination of butt, abs, and arm workouts? Don't be fooled by the slight difference in the exercise titles, such as "abs" versus "core," "twist" versus "rotation," "bridge" versus "thrust," or even "jump" versus "explode." When executed correctly, there may be a difference in these cues, but when used in a general fitness program, they are often just padding their marketing with buzz words.

In a nutshell, if you've tried a new piece of equipment or engaged in a new program in the last few decades, you've basically been doing the same program over and over again! The only essential difference is the packaging it came in, such as the program's name, instructor, exercise titles, or the location of the class.

Once you open that new package, the same problems exist: There's no assessment process to diagnose your problem and little consideration—if any at all—for how we are all very different, from our genetics to our lifestyle. There is no perfect program for all humankind even though these generalized "one-size-fits-all" programs market themselves as the answer to anyone's health and fitness problems.

For example, one person may have chronic back pain, another is just out of post-rehab for their shoulder, and another has been battling arthritis in their knees for decades. Beyond injuries, the person in front of you may be a fifty-five-year-old woman with two kids looking for time to herself, behind you a twenty-eight-year-old overweight man looking for weight loss, and to your right, a fifteen-year-old female track star looking to improve her 100-meter time, but yet you are all in the same room in the same group class, doing the same exercises. Does that really make sense?

This means you're engaging in a program that was not designed to meet your unique and idiosyncratic needs. What is more, it can't accurately track your progress and can even be exacerbating your current injuries or increasing your potential for future injury. With the understanding that lasting healthy lifestyles occur as a result of consistent progressive and healthy habit change, how can the current model of fitness ever live up to its mission statement?

This is why health and fitness professionals need to consider behavioral modification that encompasses the multidisciplinary approach to wellness, including sleep, nutrition, movement, stress, and mindset. FPs should be helping clients adopt health habits that form long-term behaviors,[33] but I think it's worth discussing how no college degree is required for any regular personal training certification.[34] Have you ever thought about the fact that the person you willingly open up to about your entire personal life, trust implicitly with your physical body, and allow them to dictate your future health status does not need to have taken even one basic anatomy course? Physical therapists, chiropractors, registered dietitians, doctors, and therapists all need multiple college degrees, followed by passing a comprehensive and rigorous board certification before they are ever able to have any influence on you or your body. So why do we not have these same kind of standards and requirements for all areas of allied healthcare, especially in a preventative powerhouse like fitness?

# Fitness Professionals Certification

In order to understand how the fitness industry has not evolved in over sixty years, we need to first grasp how the fitness industry currently regulates their professionals. Let's start with the process most personal trainers undertake to become certified since it will explain a lot about the current state of fitness.

While there is an entire comprehensive, substantive, and detailed science behind exercise, it incredibly only requires an online certification to go into practice. Not telling you how to live your life, but this fact may make you want to rethink whose program you choose to follow. Would you want to get surgery from a doctor who only

---

33    James Clear, *Atomic Habits: An Easy & Proven Way to Build Good Habits & Break Bad Ones,*1st ed. (New York: Avery, 2018).

34    National Personal Trainer Association (NPTA), "Personal Trainer Certification Requirements," https://www.personaltrainercertification.us/articles/personal-trainer-certification-requirements

spends a couple of months studying for his board exam? Oh, and what if the board exam was an online exam you could take at a general testing facility? Also, keep in mind, there is no single certification board—there are over a hundred certification companies to choose from, and all have their own approach to training. Fortunately, there are companies that are raising the bar in their standards for staff and services, but the question is how would you as a consumer know which ones they are?

Hypothetically, perhaps the gyms could take on the responsibility of sifting through who really knows their stuff and who has those top certifications. However, this would depend on what type of gym you are attending, how many trainers that gym needs to have to make a profit, what level that trainer is within the gym's hierarchy, and also how much money each customer has to spend. Even this scenario could leave you powerless to navigate your way through the fitness industry labyrinth and make progress in your own health.

## Making Change Happen

Which is why I now want to turn to expanding your understanding of how you personally can become involved in transforming the industry to ameliorate what I see as numerous injustices being perpetrated on people who are only looking to feel their best. You don't have to be powerless; in fact, the opposite is true. I think that industry-level systemic change will begin when you, the consumer, decide it's time for change. Getting off the exercise/injury hamster wheel may be as simple as applying the knowledge learned here by asking gyms more specific questions about their programs and trainers before signing up.

Supply and demand is the economic principle that underlies every legitimate and consumer-friendly business model. However, in the fitness industry, the model is exactly the opposite. The industry creates supply in order to create demand, instead of consumer demand driving what the industry supplies to meet the consumers' authentic needs. Instead, we've settled for inadequate medical care and inferior preventative care as the norm. Until recently, there has been little mention of better alternatives to preventative care. The person who said "ignorance is bliss" probably never slipped a disc after taking a group fitness class.

## CHANGE 1: PUSH FOR PREVENTION

Benjamin Franklin once said that "An ounce of prevention is worth a pound of cure." The push for prevention is the key factor to solving many of today's health issues. After all, if we can stop an illness or injury at the source, it may never happen, but it's much easier said than done to get people to accept that idea. To create this type of transformational mindset change, we would need to address such huge societal problems like how the general public currently deals with pain, the insurance industry, the healthcare system, and Big Pharma. You know, no big deal, right?

Some of these topics are beyond the scope of this book, and we aren't seeking to solve every issue here. Instead, I want to just bring your awareness to the issues at hand and the hurdles you need to overcome to get you off the exercise/injury cycle and to allow you to figure out what you need to do to maximize your results in all aspects of wellness.

Let's say I told you that you're at risk of developing migraines before you even had a slight headache—would you believe me? Or let's even assume you saw my work in person and you *do* believe me. Would you then purchase a prevention program for $100/month for three months? Or would you wait for the headaches to start and just purchase the acetaminophen for $12/bottle?

But let's say that your migraines persist for years, maybe even decades? And the $12 bottle lasts you one month with no end in sight because it only addresses the symptom rather than solving the root problem? In just three of the many years of purchasing the over-the-counter medicine, you would have spent the same amount on Tylenol that you could have spent on the three-month prevention program.

So why don't people pay for a quicker program that could actually prevent or possibly solve the problem? Why would people choose to increase their risk of liver damage that can be caused by extended use of acetaminophen[35] and still live with the pain of headaches for decades rather than engage in a program that could actually improve their health?

The answer harks back to my first question: would you trust me if you didn't have any discomfort yet? Most people would not because they assume a mentality of "If it ain't broke, don't fix it." That may be relevant in some areas of life, sure, but not health.

So even if I do a full physical assessment with you and tell you that you're at risk of a musculoskeletal injury, would you believe me? And if you did believe me, would you even want to work on it, or would you rather focus on other goals that seem more pressing at the time and worry about the injury when it happens? The answer many times is the latter, that you would wait and focus on whatever is in front of you at the moment.

So the first perspective to be shifted is how we look at our goals, which should be preventative and not "after the fact," such as someone only joining a gym when they finally accept they need to get rid of some weight. A proactive person joins a gym to prevent gaining the

---

35    Kay Brune, Bertold Renner, and Gisa Tiegs, "Acetaminophen/paracetamol: A History of Errors, Failures and False Decisions," *European Journal of Pain* (EJP) 19, no. 7 (August 2015): 953–65. https://doi.org/10.1002/ejp.621.

weight in the first place. Aesthetic goals are similar as people wait until they are "out of shape" (in either their own eyes or society's eyes) and then seek help to get "back" into shape. So then—and only then—do they turn to the fitness professional to help them solve their problem.

Besides a handful of preventative practices, the current fitness industry caters and markets toward these more immediate-feeling "quick-fix" goals because it's simple supply and demand. To see change, especially in the direction of prevention, you must start viewing *your* fitness goals differently by thinking of the future.

> **To see change ... you must start viewing your fitness goals differently by thinking of the future.**

Goals don't have to be complicated or "epic" like "I want to climb Mount Everest by this time next year." Instead, a great preventative goal can be as simple as "I want to be as strong and move as well in twenty years as I do now." Working out to be able to better play with your kids—even before you have any—is a preventative goal. Wanting to live an active lifestyle until you're well over a hundred years old is another great preventative goal.

These may seem very general, and even a little silly to some, but they are a lot wiser and realistic than a goal to lose X amount of weight in the next three months, just to put it back on in the fall and begin the same cycle over again next spring. The broad, generalized nature of these goals actually helps your fitness professional create a quality fitness program uniquely designed for you. Specifically, it helps them create a macro (at least a year-long) program for you instead of a micro (week/months) program. It's the same as consistently working on a project for months instead of waiting for the last minute and cramming everything into a few weeks.

When you see things on a macro level, you can map out how you would like to see your progress and change the plan accurately and efficiently. There's nothing wrong with being realistic by building in room for the occasional "off" day, the vacation you planned six months ago or the kid's birthday where those cupcakes from your favorite bakery are all around you. Or while we're on the topic of food, maybe you work in an office setting where someone is always bringing in donuts or bagels and cream cheese. A macro plan allows you to give yourself some grace for these circumstances rather than beating yourself up for not following an intense, short-term program perfectly.

For example, if you begin a three-month shred fat weight loss program, the person who created the program has to figure out how you can lose the most weight in three months. That's it. It is all they can focus on and there's no margin for deviation. Your past injuries, injury risk, lifestyle, time commitment, motivation, longevity, and overall health are secondary thoughts. Whereas if you give your FP a twelve-month goal or a ten-year goal, a chunk of the program can be focused around weight loss while the overall vision for the program can be centered around injury prevention and quality of life over the long term.

As I said earlier, while there are only a few preventative practices around, I'm encouraged by the growing number of trainers looking to become fitness professionals and grow their knowledge base in the direction of prevention. So if the general public transforms its mindset and increases its demand for preventative fitness services, it should make sense for the fitness industry to synchronize with that demand and supply more preventative services.

Even so, the changes to the fitness industry and the professional's training and programming would have to be vast. They would need to influence potential clients who are looking for quick fixes to see the real potential of training for longevity. Then the gyms/trainers/FPs will have to follow a new structure for programming their interventions that doesn't widely exist yet. But I think this would actually be good for the industry from a financial perspective. Instead of having to wait for the next fad exercise to promote or relying on a never-ending turnover of new customers, a solid base could be built of long-term customers committed to long-term health goals. After all, studies have shown that getting a new customer is five times more expensive for a business than keeping a current customer, not to mention that increasing customer retention by even just 5 percent can lead to profits increasing by 25–95 percent.[36] Long-term goals can lead to long-term growth.

As we discussed earlier, assessments can play a huge role in preventative fitness programming. But for now, let's talk about the programming itself. A typical high-quality program should run as follows and as originally outlined by Gray Cook.

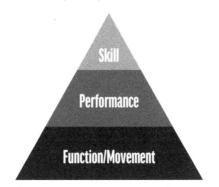

Gray Cook, 2004, *Proper Progress Demands Progressions*

The function/movement section of the pyramid forms the base because it focuses more on lifestyle movement patterns and the ability for one to complete these tasks with limited risk for injury.

---

36    Taylor Landis, "Customer Retention Marketing vs. Customer Acquisition Marketing," OutboundEngine.com, April 20, 2021, https://www.outboundengine.com/blog/customer-retention-marketing-vs-customer-acquisition-marketing/.

For example, the function/movement aspect considers things like lack of mobility, range of motion, and/or motor control. From there, you can scale up toward the performance end of fitness where you are working on physical capacity and, eventually, skill building/sport specificity at the top.

You can also think of it like the food pyramid where dessert-type items sit at the top, not because they are the most important, but because you fit them in only after other nutritional needs have been met. Likewise, skills are the dessert everybody wants to eat before the vegetables. This main meal takes more time and isn't as instantly gratifying as the dessert, but it is the healthiest and most nutritious part and should be eaten first. Our flip-flopped expectations are symptomatic of a "quick-fix" culture where we want results instantaneously, like binging on a new TV show. Remember when binging was a negative thing?

As we discussed in the QOQ Principle, functional fitness can take on many forms, but its main goal should be to improve one's form by making the person more adaptable, meaning their ability to avoid injury. If someone can't move well, it doesn't really matter how great of a coach and motivator the FP is; the lack of movement will compromise any progression. As Gray Cook says, "What is the point of exercise if we're not going to become adaptable from it? What's the point of investing your time in a movement endeavor if some capacity or competency isn't going to improve?"[37]

The general public can only respond to those questions in two ways. One is by saying the point of fitness is for aesthetics, sticking to this narrow view that they have been conditioned to believe, which avoids growth and real change. The second is that the majority of people just don't know how to engage in that type of movement or

---

37  Stuart McGill, Gray Cook, and Craig Liebenson, *Assessing Movement*.

even what Cook means when talking about movement quality, adaptability, and competency. This requires you to open up your mind to the possibility that all efforts and knowledge put forth up until this moment may have been misguided or, at the very least, lacking. This is a lot harder for most people to admit and ask, but it is what is needed for change to begin.

## CHANGE 2: CREATING TRUE PROFESSIONALS BY INCREASING REQUIREMENTS

As I see it, there is only one lasting way to solve these problems of the "quick-fix" mentality and the short-sighted goals of general fitness programs. Internally, the fitness industry needs to upgrade the standards for what qualifies somebody to be a fitness professional. This applies to everything from the information taught in certification courses to increasing the minimum requirements.

The general fitness professional will deal with clients with a wide variety of issues, goals, and needs. Making top certifications more difficult to study for and earn is one way to limit who can qualify in a way that will both increase the quality and dedication level of the professional. There are many specialty certifications currently available, such as geriatric training, working with people with disabilities, corrective exercise, sports-specific performance, and basically anything else that can get approved for certification. But this means there is a massive amount of important information missing from even the peak certifications offered by top companies like the American College of Sports Medicine (ACSM) and the National Academy of Sports Medicine (NASM). In other words, there are still thousands of dollars of educational investments and hundreds of hours more of learning before someone may be ready to professionally deal with such a diverse group of clients. Currently, these are just additional certifications one can obtain on an optional basis, but I believe the future of the industry will see the emergence of a more detailed and standardized general board certification that includes aspects of all of these.

There will continue to be underqualified people practicing fitness coaching as long as there is no national certification board administering an exam covering every topic a fitness professional needs to know in order to qualify to work in the industry. For example, in the field of nutrition, there is a clear line because of the RD exam given by the Commission of Dietetic Registration (CDR).[38] First, they require the completion of a bachelor's degree and the completion of a DPD (didactic program in dietetics) through ACEND, which is their accreditation board. After that, one must apply and get accepted, complete an ACEND-accredited dietetic internship (at least twelve hundred hours), and only then can they sit for the CDR exam. The same goes for the medical community, as they have the ACGM and AOA, and the physical therapy field, which has the ABPTS. So why the lack of board certification testing in the fitness industry?

There is no shortage of testing in the world of fitness, so a board certification should not be confused with a regular certification. There is a wide range of general certifications from thirty-minute tests you can take at your home computer to others like the ACSM exercise physiologist exam (ACSM EP-C), which requires a bachelor's degree in exercise science or a related field before you can even sit for the exam at a testing center.[39]

Beyond that, there are specialty certifications offered by top

---

38  "How to Become a Registered Dietician (RD)," Publichealthdegrees.org, accessed September 20, 2021, https://www.publichealthdegrees.org/careers/become-registered-dietitian/.

39  "Degree Requirements for the ACSM Exercise Physiologist Certification (ACSM-EP)," ACSM, https://www.acsm.org/get-stay-certified/get-certified/health-fitness-certifications/exercise-physiologist/degree-requirements-ep-c.

companies like ACSM and NASM to less-than-gold-standard (in my opinion) ones that can be earned online. So there are hundreds—if not thousands—of certifications one can get in the fitness industry, which can lead to a lot of confusion for the public on what is a quality certification. A nationally recognized board certification would provide standards and clarity that don't exist now.

One of the major reasons that something like the ACSM EP-C isn't enough to be a board certification is that it only covers topics related to exercise physiology, whereas the ideal exam should be a little wider in its scope. Since FPs see people when they are healthy and know more details about their clients' lives, an exam should include everything from advanced anatomy (including the fascial system), physiology, and biomechanics to behavior coaching, nutrition, sleep patterns, scope of practice as it pertains to these allied fitness topics, and training every type of special population, such as the elderly, children, cancer patients, and so on.

There is also the issue of creating a board of highly respected exercise and allied medical/medical professionals to review, create, and refine the exam content and the professionals it would eventually produce and be responsible for certifying. This is a lot harder to monitor, as there are thin lines as to what creates an exercise professional, but more on that later.

This certification issue is one that needs to be fixed during the first wave of improving the fitness industry, as standards dictate who FPs can help, how they can help people, and how they are viewed by the general public and other professional health communities. Remaining at today's standards will never allow us to use our potential to truly help the world. It's hard to even trust a profession where you can become certified online in as little as thirty minutes with no ongoing supervision. It's also hard to keep the standard high, as many people enter the fitness profession as a secondary job to make some money on the side or as a backup plan when they do not qualify for their nine-to-five job.

Would you want to train with somebody who is only in your gym because they couldn't get a job in finance? Would you want to train with somebody who got an online certification because they didn't want to go to college, get a degree, and study for a board exam? Would you want to go to a therapist who is a good listener but doesn't have a degree in psychology? Even most states require aspiring bartenders to go through some kind of state-mandated alcohol safety training and go through a mentorship program before they can bartend full time. But the public hears the word "certified," judges the trainer based on their "fit" appearance, and doesn't dig any deeper.

Now, this isn't to say that you still couldn't be a completely capable and qualified FP on the side if you really wanted to. Like the nutrition field, there could be a board certification and a whole process leading to the certification, but there are still millions of nutritionists who did not become an RD. Similarly, there will be fitness professionals or exercise physiologists (or an entirely new name), and there will still be the classic personal trainer. But rather than harm the industry, having higher requirements for FPs would actually be good for business. It would increase public trust, which could create higher customer loyalty, and reduce staff turnover costs for gyms and wellness centers, as certified FPs would be working in their career of choice rather than "filling time" while waiting for another opportunity.

## CHANGE 3: GENERAL PUBLIC DEMANDS BETTER SERVICE

Every major profession has evolved into better systems by implementing standard procedures. Aviation reduced pilot deaths not by increasing education, but by implementing standard cockpit proce-dures; surgery has standard procedures, and obviously the military has standard procedures. Likewise, the fitness profession needs to implement standard procedures. This can pertain to what to assess first, what assessments need to be done, proper progression tech-niques, injury prehab and rehab, and so on. Instead of being seen as "optional" services, I think these should be learned and practiced across the board.

To make that happen, the general public needs to demand a higher level of service, specifically by demanding an industry-wide list of general procedures that can be provided by a fitness professional. As stated in Change 2, a board certification would help set the guidelines for general proce-dures and a baseline as to who is a qualified FP. Then there should be an

**The general public needs to demand a higher level of service.**

established list of guidelines that all exercise professionals are required to follow as an expectation of their certification. The list could cover the gamut from the intake and assessment process to the release and completion of a client's program.

For example, in physical therapy there are specific assessments and questions a PT must ask you and perform during your intake. They must then create a personalized program based on the intake and track and submit your results to your insurance so you can continue physical therapy. Your insurance plan may give you a finite number of PT visits, but even if they didn't—or if they allot more visits than is needed—they will stop payments once a PT submits that you are not seeing much more improvement from their program. There are both benefits and drawbacks with this type of program, but the important part to focus on here is that there *is* a process, and because of that, PT is able to help millions of people every year. The process also guarantees that there are results that can then be tracked and improved upon.

While the fitness community claims to help millions of people, it's their definition of "helping" that I think is flawed. PT helps you out of pain or recover mobility, but general fitness currently just helps you lose weight, get in shape for the beach, body build, or become more athletic. These are all positive goals that many people have, but this is far from fulfilling the potential of the fitness industry. Helping people out of pain is a cause that truly changes the world, whereas getting people beach-ready is not. Helping people move better, feel better, live longer, increase their quality of life, and their ability to play with their kids is a much more compelling moral obligation that the general public needs to demand from their fitness routines. When the demand is there, it will be the industry's responsibility to supply it.

# CHAPTER 7

# Feel Better Today ... And Tomorrow

*Treatment without prevention is simply unsustainable.*
—BILL GATES

When you've been in the fitness world as long as I've been, you see the same situation happen over and over. So let's say I have a new client walk in—we'll call him Albert. He's 6'1", fifty years old, a former college football player with a mostly sedentary desk job, and he has a goal of losing thirty pounds in two months. Now, if Albert walked into most gyms, he'd get signed up to work with a trainer who would jump right into exercising, running on a treadmill, and doing box jumps.

But what I'll do with Albert before anything else is run multiple movement screens, neuromuscular patterning assessments to see what isn't functioning properly since asymmetry and imbalance, along with previous injury, are the primary predictors for pain and injury. So I'll look at Albert's gait as he walks during the exam, and perhaps I see his foot externally rotates during each step. During the squat assessment, I see his knees abduct (fall in toward the middle of his body), which indicates he could be at risk for tearing his ACL. During the assessment prescreen, I also discover he had a knee replacement twenty years before, which tells me the last thing I want to do is have him start doing box jumps and other "explosive" workouts right away.

Instead, we'll work on his balance and asymmetry issues for the first couple of weeks so that Albert doesn't become injured and quit exercise for the long run, which would cause him to ultimately gain even more weight than when he started. We would then reassess Albert, and when his screens come back with more favorable movement, then I'll feel a lot better about helping him focus on weight loss through regular exercise. We'll still keep using some of the corrective exercises since we can't fix all his problems in a couple weeks, but they can be improved enough to allow him to move more efficiently and ensure his imbalance doesn't resurface. So it might end up taking him four months to lose the weight instead of the two he had planned for, but he's going to feel a lot better while doing it and be able to meet his goal, which he won't be able to do if he lands in the doctor's office two weeks later and then has a procedure followed by eight weeks of physical therapy.

As I see it, there are really only three possibilities when you set goals for an exercise program:

- Work on improving the short term

- Work on improving the long term

- A mix of both

Working on short-term goals tends to be the common focal point as best seen in the popular weight-loss and aesthetics programs currently available to the public, while a long-term approach like living longer, having less pain as you age, and reducing your injury risk are discussed much less.

Now the mix of the two is where you can set a *micro* and *macro* goal. Your micro goal can be your short-term weight loss for a summer body, while having a long-term plan to feel better would extend over the next decade. That plan can have macro programs where weight loss is one of a couple of your main areas of focus around the spring months, but perhaps during the other nine months, you can consider movement, technique, and healthcare as your major areas of focus. One of the great benefits of a program like this is that the micro goals (losing weight) can be seen as natural results of the macro goals (feel better).

To play devil's advocate, an argument to be made against this multifaceted type of approach is the overlapping principle. While a short-term goal like weight loss is primarily just set for an outcome in a few months, one can argue those results last much further into the future. If you do a high-intensity program, you are still putting your body into a positive eustress that will cause adaptation in your physical self that will last beyond those few months and even when the weight is regained.

The argument can also be made for only having a macro program. If you have a macro goal like improving your quality of movement slowly throughout the rest of your life, you can't reach those goals without, even unintentionally, having micro goals too. To improve your movement long term, you have to start somewhere. Again, for either program you would need an assessment, but afterward, even if your goal was highly aspirational, such as "continuous improvement for the rest of your life," your assessment would reveal aspects of your movement to begin focusing as your first micro goals within your macro program.

A real mix would be long-term goals supported by short-term goals. For example, let's say your macro/long-term goal is to have "better quality of movement." That may be supported by a set of micro/short-term goals that include things like weight loss over the first six months or being able to run a 5K. The micro goal and the macro goals here don't directly correlate, but they can both be worked effectively into the same program without contradicting one another. The difference is that you forgo the hardcore push for weight loss (i.e., dropping thirty pounds in three months or less) to a slightly lengthier but more focused six-month weight loss program, which allows you to work on weight loss without sacrificing the movement quality and still make progress on both fronts.

The issue that prevents this type of new mindset shift from sweeping the industry isn't that the general public can't understand the differences, it's that these types of mixes of long-term and short-term goals would require an entirely new type of professional than what is currently present in the marketplace. So before you can set goals and seek help, and even before you go out and find a fitness professional who fits your needs (and your new mentality toward health and longevity), you need to understand the potential risk for injury involved in short-term programs. Moreover, you need to understand the risk of using a trainer who isn't adequately educated in fitness and wellness.

# Health and Injury Risk Reduction Continuum (HIRRC)

Let us begin to narrow our focus more on the exercise industry's approach at improving one's quality of life and not just their short-term goals. Instead of trying to fix people's pain, we need to be more concerned with stopping it *before* it starts. To be truly successful, prevention practices will require the involvement of all fields, but I believe the fitness community can take the lead because we are the ones that not only see you when you are healthy, but are also not limited by insurance protocols. This leaves the fitness industry free to set the rules, so to speak, but the downside to this freedom is that it has allowed the industry to run *too* freely and not maintain any sort of quality control, like we discussed before.

> Instead of trying to fix people's pain, we need to be more concerned with stopping it before it starts.

This is a burden that the fitness industry should be helping to bear, but it ends up falling mostly on the general public's health statistics. In Part 4, we will cover how you can start to navigate through this seemingly complex, constantly evolving field of fitness, allowing you to be ahead of the changes that may take the industry decades to make and keep you safe while pursuing your fitness goals. To fully comprehend the multitude of choices available to you, we'll start with an explanation of how the industry is progressing and the general idea of the new fitness professional.

Since fitness professionals range from part-time trainers with no strong educational background to exercise physiologists with doctorates in exercise science, I've developed the Health/Injury Risk Reduction (HIRRC) Model to take you through the first step of understanding the new paradigm shift. This model and the prehab/rehab scale (explained in the next chapter) are the outlines to the future of fitness.

Frankly, the industry just isn't up-to-date in how we communicate with the public, and we need to be doing a better job at helping the public understand the difference between the different types of fitness professionals out there so you know which one to pursue, whether a general trainer, a corrective specialist, an exercise physiologist, or an athletic performance coach.

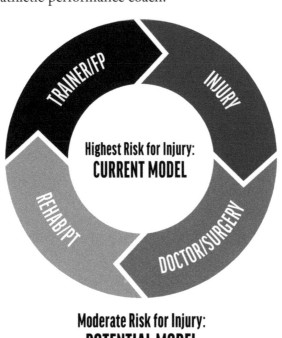

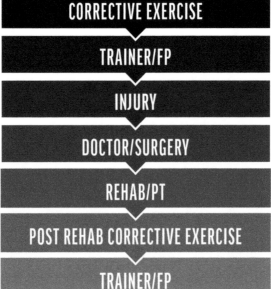

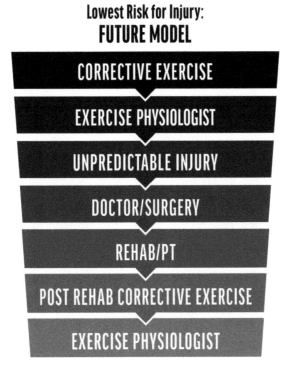

Lowest Risk for Injury:
FUTURE MODEL

CORRECTIVE EXERCISE

EXERCISE PHYSIOLOGIST

UNPREDICTABLE INJURY

DOCTOR/SURGERY

REHAB/PT

POST REHAB CORRECTIVE EXERCISE

EXERCISE PHYSIOLOGIST

In today's fitness industry, you'll mostly find certified personal trainers along with unintended consequences of exercise training, such as injury caused *by* exercise.[40] It is not that these two are always correlated, but exercise is now seen as a potential risk factor for injury instead of being a factor for *lessening* one's injury risk. Although it is difficult to determine the exact percentages or the precise causes, some of the common risk factors I've seen are the following:

- Exercise quantity (overexercising), particularly in deconditioned individuals (those who have lost fitness through lack of exercise)
- Improper use of equipment
- Previous history of injury

40  Harold Kohl III and Tinker Murray, *Foundations of Physical Activity and Public Health*, 1st ed. (Champaign, IL: Human Kinetics, 2012).

With this last one, there is also a consideration regarding the type of injury, including both noncontact and contact injuries. Implementing certain movement assessments may be a key to potentially understanding increased risk of injury.[41] As discussed before, the future model will be designed to produce the lowest risk for injury, but only once the bar is raised and the standard fitness professional is required to be an exercise physiologist (EP) and EPs are all certified in corrective exercise. This will happen because the EP will routinely screen for injury risks, along with a myriad of other tests, and then analyze results to create a program that will not only improve the client's weight or aesthetic goals, but will improve their overall life quality as well. Don't worry—we will go through how to navigate the industry to find an EP or truly qualified FP in the last couple of chapters.

Until the future model is effectuated, we still have the option to find a workable alternative within the current model. If you are not lucky enough to find an EP who is certified in corrective exercise today, you can always find a corrective exercise specialist at almost any top gym around the country. From there, once you have worked thoroughly with this professional, you can move to a personal trainer to continue to work more closely on your aesthetic or weight loss goals.

Seeing the corrective exercise specialist first will already improve your function and reduce your risk of injury. But due to higher prices charged by these specialists and the fact that they will usually want

---

41    Scott E. Landis, Russell T. Baker, and Jeff G. Seegmiller, "Non-contact Anterior Cruciate Ligament and Lower Extremity Injury Risk Prediction Using Functional Movement Screen and Knee Abduction Moment: An Epidemiological Observation of Female Intercollegiate Athletes," *The International Journal of Sports Physical Therapy* 13, no. 6 (December 2018): 973, https://doi.org/10.26603/ijspt20180973; Emma Moore, Samuel Chalmers, Steve Milanese, and Joel T. Fuller, "Factors Influencing the Relationship Between the Functional Movement Screen and Injury Risk in Sporting Populations: A Systematic Review and Meta-analysis," *Sports Medicine* 49 (2019): 1449–63, https://doi.org/10.1007/s40279-019-01126-5.

to take a slower pace to the aesthetics goals than what the general public is used to, a personal trainer will often be most people's next move since the general perception is a personal trainer will speed up the process of achieving their aesthetic goals—and at a lower cost. But the important thing you should remember is that even if you are paying more in the beginning, it will save you money in the long run because injuries are far from cheap.[42]

To go back to my client Albert, if he works with a standard-issue personal trainer at his local gym doing high intensity workouts without correcting his balance issues or considering his past injury history, it wouldn't surprise me if he ends up tearing his ACL, goes to the doctor, has surgery, and then spends weeks—maybe even months—before he can even go on a walk around his neighborhood again, much less get back into the gym. Which route was really cheaper in the end?

At that point, he could also decide "The heck with it!" and abandon exercise altogether because he feels he will just get hurt again. It's not farfetched to think that even a short amount of time on the E/I Cycle would make many people decide they would rather be overweight than limping along, in and out of surgery, and racking up medical bills.

## The Annual Checkup

There are two new concepts that, if put into practical motion, can change the way the whole world feels, moves, and understands their own bodies. The first is that you, the public, should be setting up annual checkups, not just with your doctor, but with your fitness professional who knows you and sees you. Most people only get a checkup

---

42   "Physical Therapy Cost," Thervo.com, accessed July 10, 2021, https://thervo.com/costs/physical-therapy-cost.

from an allied health or health professional after being injured. But the easiest way to avoid injury, even if you're not currently active in exercising, is to set up an annual checkup/assessment.

Ideally, you'd see an exercise physiologist (EP) who is also certified in corrective exercise and has a background in physical therapy. They would assess you for movement quality, pain evaluations, and risks for potential injury. You might wonder how this is different from your annual physical with your primary care physician (PCP), but you have to remember that the point is that your EP is more familiar with you, seeing you more often than your PCP, and can interpret your results from a fitness perspective, not just an internist perspective.

Also, the fact that certain checkups are called "physicals" can be very misleading. Yes, they will be doing various tests to see how your body is functioning internally, but they do not test for movement quality, risk for injury, and the quality of your lifestyle through movement that I'm referring to as a functional movement physical. Think of it like this: Even if you have an annual physical, you still go to your dentist for follow-ups because the physical doesn't cover that part of the body. You want to catch cavities before they require a root canal, right? Likewise, your annual physical may not include all aspects of your body like your muscles, joint function, neuromuscular cohesiveness, and more, which an EP will pay attention to.

As we move into a world of preventative medicine and health-care, we need to look at what testing will be done to set the baseline. In terms of movement professionals (FPs, PTs, OTs, etc.), the fitness professional stands as the best equipped to take on the task of annually assessing the general public. Again, I'm talking about specifically qualified and very well educated fitness professionals who have regular contact with their clients, approach them with a pre-ventative mindset, are trained in quality of movement, and are the freest (in terms of involvement with insurance) to design a new way of conducting annual assessments. Even if insurance becomes a part of the fitness world and can be used for annual assessments, the new FPs will already be able to design the process and dictate how it will work, not the other way around.

Eighty percent of the American population doesn't belong to a gym,[43] but annual assessments could benefit even those who do not want to join a gym and those who do not want to use a trainer—or even exercise in general. In my experience, most people don't like going to the doctor, and even fewer people like going to their dentist, but since many people don't floss daily like they should, the annual checkup serves as a protective barrier to get things back on track from any unhealthy habits. Likewise, an annual assessment would allow you to live your life pretty much as you please, while also being alerted to the major flaws in your lifestyle, even the ones that may be deadly. After all, if it weren't for recommended physicals, the rate of obesity, heart disease, diabetes, oral cancer, gum disease, and more would be even higher.

From a business perspective, a gym offering holistic annual physicals would have a new way to generate revenue from people who would normally never walk through their doors. Some of those visits could then translate into new customers, new services, and additional revenue that doesn't involve personal trainers harassing current customers who are just trying to get in a few minutes on the treadmill before they have to go sit in an office all day. Now, a quick note: these fitness checkups are by no means meant to replace your annual physical with a PCP, as they will look for things that an EP wouldn't be able to assess or diagnose. Rather, it's meant to be complementary

---

43   "Gym Market Research & Industry Stats 2020," Wellness Creative Co, July 1, 2020, https://www.wellnesscreatives.com/gym-market-statistics/.

to the annual physical and help someone have a more holistic view of themselves and their fitness needs.

Imagine what a fitness checkup could do to the world's health statistics. Besides the individual improvements like that of movement quality, lifestyle, and longevity, the societal rates of disease that healthcare checkups are designed to identify would also decline. Improving one's movement and fitness habits, while also covering their overall nutrition, sleep, and regeneration (with the ability to refer out to a specialist if necessary), would directly impact and lower a person's risk of those same healthcare concerns like heart disease, diabetes, and obesity. The fitness checkup could surprise the world as the most important appointment of them all.

# Kinesiological Quotient (KQ)

Now let's discuss a topic so important that I think it deserves its own book. We just discussed how an annual checkup for movement and fitness is of utmost importance. Just as Gray Cook did when he created the functional movement screen (FMS), we need to put numbers and standards to these assessments and then possibly use those assessments to look more broadly at health across the world. What if we could set up a standard of physical function/movement tests that can be taken to generate a numbered outcome which could then be compared to that of everybody else in the world? Similar to an intelligence quotient (IQ), or the newly recognized emotional quotient (EQ), a kinesiological quotient (KQ) could prove to be a parallel measure to validate the

> We must try to understand our bodies in terms of movement as much as we try to understand our brains.

benefits of fitness. We must try to understand our bodies in terms of movement as much as we try to understand our brains.

When looking at a child who is trying out for a sports team, understanding their current KQ could help determine whether or not they are physically ready for a specific sport. When a person wants to start an exercise program, a KQ would give the FP a baseline for understanding their readiness for fitness. KQ could help determine if athletes are built or born—or both. Even more broadly, we can use KQ to direct those who may need more movement-based training in the proper direction and use it as a guide to prescribe programs. The data could even be used to compare the levels of different countries to see how different lifestyles across the world determine their populations, health, injury, and movement outcomes. Furthermore, it can be used to pinpoint further improvements in the industry—what works, what doesn't, even specific trends for different demographics.

I'm not saying that IQ or EQ are perfect evaluations of one's intellectual or emotional intelligence, but they do serve as a great baseline that is widely recognized. For example, intelligence can be defined in many ways: the financial success of a person, the grades they achieved and the universities they attended, the way they are able to navigate around their external environment, their ability to pick up a new skill or trade, and more. So even if IQ doesn't directly predict who will have a large impact on the world, it still allows us to have a marker to look back on and compare them to the world today. The tests have even changed, improved, and diversified throughout the years, but the idea that IQ may be a strong marker of intelligence still remains a common strategy to help guide one's educational needs. If this is true for IQ, what can KQ tell us?

What can it tell us about history? Would we be able to compare athletes today to the warriors or gladiators of the Roman Empire?

Can we further understand why height differentials and quality of movement differ from people across nations? Would we be able to show a decline in movement quality in our children as they progress through the sedentary school system? The areas where KQ could be applied are endless. Again, it is by no means meant to be the end-all be-all, but another marker or tool to help us understand ourselves—and more importantly, how to improve ourselves.

If somebody has a low KQ, it doesn't mean they can never be an athlete, just as somebody with a low IQ can still become very successful. A person with a low EQ isn't destined to be socially awkward, but it shows that they may need to focus on developing skills by increasing their social interaction or by working with a behavioral therapist. Without understanding their EQ, they may have never known they were missing those social skills. KQ would be no different, and the importance of having a widely recognized standard test for fitness and health should be as clear as that of IQ and EQ.

Until the industry fully accepts these ideas and moves in this direction, my practical advice to avoid injury immediately is ask good questions, look at things with a long-term perspective, and seek out an FP—or EP—who understands corrective exercise and can set you up for success in your fitness goals by examining the best way to keep you off the E/I Cycle and get you on the right track to moving better, feeling better, and living longer. Trust me, there are a lot of Alberts—and Albertas—out there, so you're not alone, and with the right fitness professional, you don't have to stay alone.

# CHAPTER 8

# Looks Aren't Everything

*Never judge someone by the way he looks or a book by the way it's covered; For inside those tattered pages, there's a lot to be discovered.*
—STEPHEN COSGROVE

If you've ever seen the movie *Back to the Future III*, you might recall that the majority of the action is set in 1885 in Wild West California. In one scene, a character reveals he's from the future and starts sharing with a confused audience of ranchers and farmers all the inventions and changes that are to come. When he's asked what people do for fun in the future, he responds by listing a series of hobbies, including running. This further confuses his audience, who can't imagine why anyone in their right mind would run "for fun."

But the scene couldn't be more right. While athletics and competitive sports have been around for most of recorded human history, the idea of needing fitness for health or as a recreational activity is still a very new idea. After all, humankind has evolved from being hunter-gatherers to our sedentary modern jobs. And you can see a clear correlation between early athletic challenges (archery, javelin, running) with the practical needs of human society (hunting/gathering).

When you're living a nomadic lifestyle or working on the farm all day, you will probably stay "in shape" without really trying. But with the Industrial Revolution and the Tech Boom, we not only no longer move the same way, but we don't expend the same amount of calories per day or exercise the same muscles in a functional way. This has helped create the fitness industry that we know as these cultural and lifestyle changes have caused changes in our overall health.

The three mainstream avenues of fitness—or "genres" of fitness, if you like—that have dominated the industry for almost a century are weight loss, athletics, and bodybuilding/aesthetics. But with the new age of fitness come new types of fitness professionals and therefore new practices. Fitness is beginning to intertwine more and more with healthcare. While this evolution has been a long time coming, fitness still needs strong change agents in order to meet its full potential of becoming an allied health field.

As we've already discussed, exercise physiologists are generally considered to be the top fitness professionals; however, the problem is that most of their education is in current health fields like cardiac rehabilitation. Although this is an extremely important area of healthcare, and while EPS' commitment to higher learning is commendable, I believe they have missed the areas of healthcare that most of us need.

By way of analogy, the reason a registered dietitian is seen and needed as an allied medical professional is not only because of the rigorous education process, but because nutrition plays such a large and obvious role in healthcare. The same can be said for movement. There's a popular saying used for weight loss that goes "You can't out-train a bad diet."[44] This means no matter how hard you exercise, you can't lose weight if you're eating too many calories. It emphasizes the importance of nutrition in an exercise program, but it also undervalues the importance of movement in one's health practices. The saying has been made popular by the fitness industry as they push their weight-loss nutrition programs, so it's easy to see the irony and, more importantly, the problem with this type of myopic and unidimensional thinking.

Exercise in this example is seen only as a way to help aid weight loss. When the fitness industry dismisses exercise as an equally important component and pigeonholes movement into being only a tool for calorie burning, it shifts the public's view of the potential and the goals of the fitness industry. Just as you can't out-train a bad diet, you also can't outlive poor movement. Longevity and the quality of that longevity is based directly on one's ability to live one's life easily and happily. Indeed, if you can't move well, you can't live well either.

The HIRRC is a great outline to explain the new breed of fitness professional, and as we move more toward exercise physiologists dominating the field, the available specialties (i.e., geriatric, pediatric, disabilities, etc.) will begin to change as well. These specialties are relatively new but are rapidly expanding and gaining more validity through the field of exercise science as the public learns to better advocate for their needs. After all, a specialized fitness program for a twelve-year-old who just got diagnosed with Type 1 diabetes will need to be very different than a program for a forty-five-year-old undergoing chemotherapy. Therefore, it's essential to truly understand the necessity of these emerging professions. Luckily, once you begin to learn more about them, their value becomes clearer.

---

44    Aseem Malhotra, Timothy Noakes, and Stephen Phinney, "It is Time to Bust the Myth of Physical Inactivity and Obesity: You Cannot Outrun a Bad Diet," *British Journal of Sports Medicine* 49, no. 15 ( August 2015), https://doi.org/10.1136/bjsports-2015-094911.

The most commonly used new practice is called "corrective exercise," or prehabilitation (prehab). This is where a person is evaluated for movement quality, as well as risks for potential injury.[45] Following this evaluation, specific exercise prescriptions are utilized to lower the risk of injury before a person begins training. At minimum, these results are applied in the beginning of a person's exercise program, as prescribed in the low-injury risk HIRRC model.

In the new fitness exercise field, the exercise physiologist (EP), or corrective exercise specialist (CES), will also understand their scope of practice better, which will begin to ameliorate the E/I Cycle. Once injury occurs during any point of an exercise program or daily life, there must be rehabilitation, and the EP would know when this occurs or when an assessment shows the person needs to be referred out. At this point, an orthopedist, physical therapist, or chiropractor will then evaluate and treat the acute injury or repair from recent surgery.

Once released from rehab, there are several available options such as take-home exercises to continue the same program on your own at home or open-gym concepts where you can do your exercises at the physical therapy clinic without direct supervision of the physical therapist. Most people do not choose to do open-gym exercise, and less people do their take-home exercises recommended by their PT. Even if they do, it's important to note that even take-home exercises will need to be progressed after at least four to six (at most eight) weeks of continuous execution. This is where an FP or EP with a knowledge of PT—and ideally, some communication with the PT—can help structure a long-term program for long-term progress.

This scenario creates the next area for a trained fitness professional to step in, and that is for post-rehabilitation training. Post-

---

45   NASM, *Essentials of Corrective Exercise Training*, 1st revised ed. (Burlington, MA: Jones & Bartlett Learning, 2013).

rehab happens upon completion of a rehab program and involves different evaluations that allow the client's program to be progressed accordingly. The goal of a post-rehab program is not simply to get them back to basic daily functioning, but to have the client exceed their rehabilitation goals.

For example, imagine a person completes rehab for a herniated disc in their cervical spine and feels 100 percent better in their daily life at the time of discharge. But then they have recurring neck pain when they go to lift their grandkids, sit for too long, or return to playing sports. In such a situation, they are not fully recovered. The best way to get back to a fully active lifestyle is to complete a post-rehabilitation program. This practice should be routinely taught in detail to every EP, letting them decide in which specific EP domain they would like to specialize.

These same two ends of pre/rehabilitation extend beyond just orthopedics and musculoskeletal injury. Prehab and post-rehab also apply to cardiovascular health and disease. Prevention is still the key here as well, but once there is a cardiovascular problem and intervention is needed, a strong post-rehabilitation program is the most important practice that will get you back to living the life you desire. This is why learning how to distinguish not only who are the right professionals, but when to go see one is critical to taking back control of your health and wellness.

First, we cover and outline the different types of professionals and present an easy-to-navigate tool to help you recognize the differences so you can readily distinguish among them. The hardest part about getting involved in fitness and knowing how to get off the E/I Cycle is where you should start, so we'll share some baseline examples to help you identify where you might fall on the cycle.

# FITNESS STAGE SCALE
## *No gains until there's no pain*

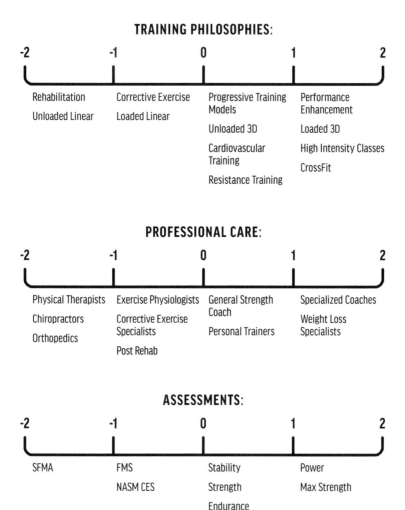

### TRAINING PHILOSOPHIES:

-2        -1        0        1        2

| -2 | -1 | 0 | 1 |
|---|---|---|---|
| Rehabilitation | Corrective Exercise | Progressive Training Models | Performance Enhancement |
| Unloaded Linear | Loaded Linear | Unloaded 3D | Loaded 3D |
| | | Cardiovascular Training | High Intensity Classes |
| | | Resistance Training | CrossFit |

### PROFESSIONAL CARE:

-2        -1        0        1        2

| -2 | -1 | 0 | 1 |
|---|---|---|---|
| Physical Therapists | Exercise Physiologists | General Strength Coach | Specialized Coaches |
| Chiropractors | Corrective Exercise Specialists | Personal Trainers | Weight Loss Specialists |
| Orthopedics | Post Rehab | | |

### ASSESSMENTS:

-2        -1        0        1        2

| -2 | -1 | 0 | 1 |
|---|---|---|---|
| SFMA | FMS | Stability | Power |
| | NASM CES | Strength | Max Strength |
| | | Endurance | |

If you are currently in pain, you will need to see a rehabilitation specialist such as a physical therapist, chiropractor, or orthopedic doctor depending on your issue. The fitness stage scale above is a Likert-type scale from -2 to 2, so this would put you at a -2. Once you receive the rehab and are released, it's time for post-rehabilitation, which places you at a -1. Meanwhile, 0 represents that you're not injured but also not engaged in a fitness program. 0 is your baseline, so even post-rehab means you're not ready for general function or growth work just yet.

The 0 level applies to anyone who completed rehab and post-rehab, or anyone who is not injured but looking to start a fitness program. Level 1 is for your moderate fitness enthusiast, and 2 is for your die-hard exercise enthusiast or athlete.

It's important to understand that this is a sliding scale. For example, once an athlete retires, they should not fall to a 0, but a 1. If they got injured, they would fall from a 2 to a -2 immediately, but if they retired due to numerous injuries, their program may need to fluctuate between a -1 to 1 for the rest of their life.

The average person will probably fall at 0 or -1 depending on training philosophies that each professional will follow at each different number on the scale. For example, -2 is targeted at rehabilitation professionals, and therefore their training philosophies will dictate utilizing unloaded (no added weight or even reducing body weight) linear or single joint movements. Examples of these type of exercises are glute bridges, ball kick-outs, shoulder external rotation.

Once you move from a -2 to a -1, you are closer to baseline. Your pain is relieved and therefore you can do more advanced movements, but you still have a short journey before you can be back at a 0. So here you would see your exercise physiologist who specializes in post-rehabilitation. You can even find one that specializes in corrective exercises, but in either case, you would have to make sure they understand your previous injury and the rehabilitation program you just completed. You would not be ready to go see a trainer or work on goals like weight loss or aesthetics just yet.

You're ready to train for weight loss or aesthetics once you graduate from -1 and move to a 0. As discouraging as it can feel to be called a 0 after completing all that hard work, it's again only meant to express that you aren't quite ready for advanced movements. But here you can begin to see a general trainer or strength coach. Your body has now been realigned, stabilized, mobilized, and is ready for your more athletic or aesthetic goals. However, it still needs to be taken at a slower pace. At this stage, you would want to look for a professional whose training philosophies are more unloaded three-dimensional movements, slight strength and cardiovascular training, and a slow progressing exercise program. In other words, you're not ready just yet for training for the local triathlon.

Once Phase 1 moves toward 2, you can step up your game. You don't need to be an athlete or have athletic goals to move toward a 2. This level would also include your high-intensity workouts, loaded three-dimensional movement training, Olympic-style lifting, and—if you're looking for it—programs like CrossFit.

To make it easier to figure out what I'm talking about here, I've also developed a four-quadrant model below, which is just another way to look at the fitness stage scale above:

## PREHAB/REHAB 4 QUADRANTS

2 Axes:

- **Y Axis:** Movement Professionals - Specialists
- **X Axis:** Pain/Injury - No Pain/Injury

4 Quadrants:

- **Upper Left:** Movement Specialists focusing on Pain management
- **Upper Right:** General Health Coaches and Personal Trainers
- **Bottom Left:** Clinical Pain Specialists: Physical Therapists and Chiropractors

- **Bottom Right:** Specialty Coaches (ex.: Sport Specific Coaches and Extreme Weight Loss Coaches)

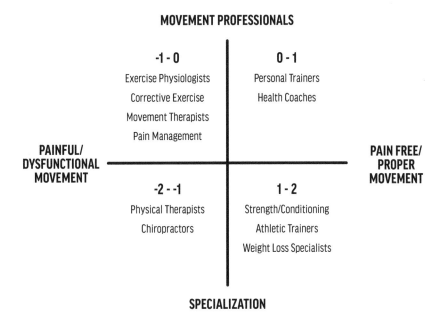

This model also uses the -2 to 2 levels to show where you currently may fall and what exercises/training styles you will be experiencing at each level. Whichever you prefer, both charts show the importance of scaling up a program and expose the common problems that could lead to injury or reinjury.

If you are a -1 and you engage in a popular high-intensity weight loss program, you are jumping too many levels since you haven't completed the prerequisites for engaging in that type of activity. You would be moving from corrective, linear exercises to weighted explosive three-dimensional movements. Hopefully by now, you can see how a body that is barely ready for learning a basic squat pattern is far from ready to do weighted jump squats onto a plyo box.

As shown in the pre/rehab four quadrants, weight loss is a 1–2 level exercise, but exercise professionals are needed from a -2 all the way to a 2. Thus, the chart emphasizes how fitness in this new age will span way beyond just weight loss and aesthetics. I believe the world of healthcare needs our help, but also because a new type of professional must arise to get the general population ready for this type of training. The current fitness industry that keeps pushing weight loss simply is not equipped for it.

As a side note, although a fitness professional is not listed in the -2 stages, they are often aids. If they are not, they still need to be well versed in the rehabilitation fields, and that's why it falls on the scale. Even your level 2 coach needs to have some sort of education in -2 since the number one predictor for injury is previous injury[46] and our bodies rarely heal back to 100 percent after an injury. For example, if you sprain your ankle, chronic instability may result despite being able to resume normal activities.[47] Therefore, your level 2 coach needs to not only be aware of your injury but also equipped with the tools to adapt your program in a way that will prevent reinjury.

This is why education of the new fitness professional needs to span all levels and why every level needs its own specialists. Without the corrective exercise professional and the post-rehab exercise physiologist, the general population will never be able to get off the E/I Cycle, and it will largely be the fault of the exercise industry. However, it's your responsibility to seek out the professionals who teach at your current level, which we will dive into more in Part 4, but you must understand the differences between each type of professional and know which one to look for at each stage of your fitness journey.

---

46  Gray Cook, *Athletic Body in Balance.*

47  Carl G. Mattacola and Maureen K. Dwyer, "Rehabilitation of the Ankle After Acute Sprain or Chronic Instability," *Journal of Athletic Training* 37, no. 4 (2002): 413–29, https://www.ncbi.nlm.nih.gov/pmc/articles/PMC164373/; Lars Konradsen, Susanne Olesen, and Henrik M. Hansen, "Ankle Sensorimotor Control and Eversion Strength after Acute Ankle Inversion Injuries," *American Journal of Sports Medicine* 26, no. 1 (1998): 72–77, https://doi.org/10.1177/03635465980260013001.

Ideally, the FP of the future will prescribe the right person for you at each stage, but until the industry is mature enough to help you make this distinction, you will need to take control of your search.

When you set a goal of avoiding injury and feeling better, aesthetics and weight loss should naturally follow, so even if you don't have a certified EP in your area, this can help you initiate the conversation with a trainer on what you really need and want out of a program. No matter what "genre" of fitness you are pursuing or where you fall from -2 to 2, my hope is that these tools can at least help you be more strategic in how you view your past level of fitness, realistically assess your present state, and pursue your future state of fitness.

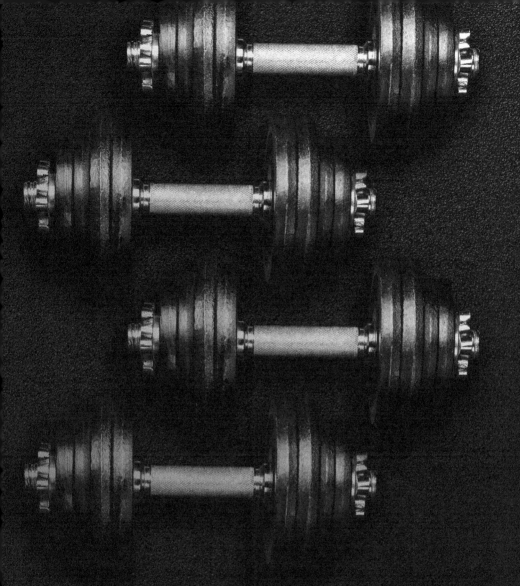

**PART 4:**

# Navigating to Victory

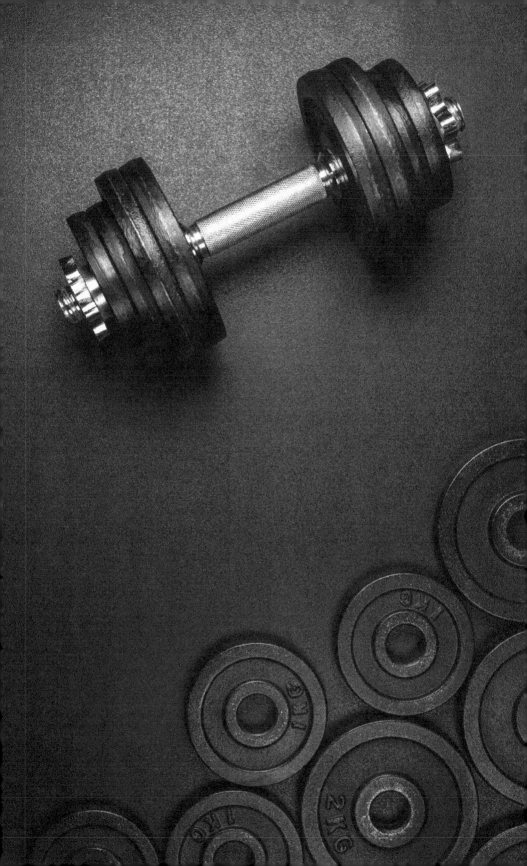

CHAPTER 9

# Let's Get Deep

*The will to win, the desire to succeed, the urge to*
*reach your full potential ... these are the keys that*
*will unlock the door to personal excellence.*
—CONFUCIUS

In 2017, I was asked to speak in front of medical professionals from the largest health system—and employer for that matter—in all of New York state. This was to be a series of talks, part of a larger wellness initiative. My first topic was "The Benefits of Prehabilitation," and looking back, it was no wonder not many people signed up. At the time, I don't think most people even understood the word.

I realized the major problem was the message. People wanted to follow the culture; they wanted a quick fix. So I changed the title of the next lecture to "Achieving Real Results in Your Workout Program." It was my way of still sticking to my morals but seeing if rephrasing the title would create more interest by meeting people where they were.

Every seat was signed up for the day the email was blasted out. Same lecture, different title. I was ecstatic to have a large audience to share my knowledge of finding the right professional, the importance of prehab in an exercise program, and how to view fitness as a lifelong goal. The big day came, and I set up all the chairs in perfect rows throughout my fitness studio. If you've never seen a gym being set up for a conference, it's definitely a sight to behold. Chairs peeked out from behind large cable pulley machines with enough room between each for the participant to demo exercises, but not too far where they would feel isolated from each other. Let's just say it's not a typical classroom setup. But I didn't care—I would put chairs on my treadmills if it meant I could reach more ears. And to top it off, these were *medical* professionals—doctors, nurses, and physician assistants, all the way to administrators for the health system, the people who make policy for the hospital!

I wore my nice mix of professional and fitness clothes: stretchy black dress pants with a colored, not too tightly fitting exercise Henley shirt. My slides were up, everybody was seated, my nerves were exploding, and I was ready to begin. About three minutes into my introduction, I saw a sea of blank faces. An internal panic started to wash over me, and I was pretty sure the audience was beginning to notice.

"Am I not exciting enough? Should I be smiling more? Should I have started with a story?" were all questions I began to ask myself.

I continued on, and it all became clear around the five-minute mark when a nurse raised her hand and asked, "Yeah, okay, but I've been told my BMI (body mass index) is too high, so will any of these exercises help me lose some weight now?"

I was floored, and I'm pretty sure my mouth was open for a couple of seconds because half of the audience began to lean in as they awaited my response. How do you tell a crowd of medical professionals that they have completely missed the point of the way to see their own health? Not to mention my stupidity in taking a question in the first five minutes of a sixty-minute presentation. Her question would have been somewhat addressed as the hour continued, but now I needed to sum it up on the spot.

I responded, "Who told you your BMI is too high?"

She simply responded, "My doctor."

To which I replied, "And what was their follow-up to that statement?"

She looked at me as if I was trying to avoid her question or embarrass her, as if the answer seemed so obvious. With a bit of annoyance in her voice, she said, "Start exercising."

So I continued, "Exercise where?"

She shrugged and said, "I don't know, anywhere?"

I asked, "Okay, exercise with whom?"

Again, she just shrugged. Little did I realize at the time that those questions would lead me into a series of talks on just the answer to those questions alone.

The takeaway from the story is that external motivation is just that—external. Somebody or something else pushing you to learn more about fitness. The fact that most of the audience was more engaged at that moment showed how strong *external* forces were in motivating people to exercise, even in the medical field. The problem is that it was all for the wrong reasons. That nurse had no plans to begin an exercise routine until her doctor mentioned it. She was then given no direction as to how to start or accomplish a proper fitness program. She had no *internal* drive to partake in the real definition of fitness; she just wanted a quick "Band-Aid" or easy 1-2-3 steps for weight loss to fix what her doctor diagnosed as a "weight issue."

Intrinsic or internal motivation is a different driver. It's the driver that allows founders to create world-changing companies, scientists to develop life-saving drugs, and even for me as a movement professional to sit at a computer on and off for years to share what I've learned.

> You must be the one who decides to make a change or move in a new direction; it cannot be your doctor, your family, or even your spouse's decision for you.

Internal motivation doesn't always need to be connected to passion. Sometimes the motivation is just because you understand engaging in the activity will improve your life. It doesn't mean you are passionate about it or have a drive to complete a certain task; it's just a self-awareness that it's a necessity. You must be the one who decides to make a change or move in a new direction; it cannot be your doctor, your family, or even your spouse's decision for you. Once you have the internal drive to accomplish a specific goal, I think there is very little that can stop you.

## Who Are You Doing This For?

In order to understand the reasons why individuals begin or continue physical activity, one must consider the perspective of self-determination theory (SDT),[48] which is impacted by several types of motivation, including extrinsic and intrinsic.

---

48   Richard M. Ryan and Edward L. Deci, *Self-Determination Theory: Basic Psychological Needs in Motivation, Development, and Wellness*, 1st ed. (New York: The Guilford Press, 2018); Manuel Jacob Sierra-Díaz, Sixto González-Víllora, Juan Carlos Pastor-Vicedo, and Guillermo López-Sánchez, "Can We Motivate Students to Practice Physical Activities and Sports Through Models-Based Practice? A Systematic Review and Meta-Analysis of Psychosocial Factors Related to Physical Education," *Frontiers in Psychology* 10 (2019): 2115, https://doi.org/10.3389/fpsyg.2019.02115.

Extrinsic motivation is influenced by something external and consumes us on a daily basis, such as losing weight, running a marathon, making more money, or wanting to look like a goddess. In fact, messages are sent constantly from advertisers reflecting beautiful fitness models on the front pages of websites, social media pages, and magazines because of the potential influence they may possess. They are also reflected in your family and friends telling you that you need to get in shape or lose weight to the point you internalize these messages as you set your fitness goals but only because you want to look a certain way for your friends or followers while strutting on the beach. This is the essence of extrinsic, or what we like to call external motivations.

In my experience, however, real change hardly ever starts from external motivation. Tony Robbins teaches a concept that internal motivation *pulls* you to your goals, while external motivation *pushes* you. It's much easier to get to where you're going if you feel pulled instead of pushed.

I'd say most people start an exercise program due to some sort of external motivation. Far too often it takes a major trauma, illness, or injury in somebody's life for them to gain the internal wake-up call to start exercising. It may be easier to convince yourself to start an exercise program once you've reached an age where you can't walk up a flight of stairs as easily as you once did or be able to play on the ground with your kids. Many people start an exercise program once they've reached a breaking point in their weight and they hate what they see when they look in the mirror or when they receive a diagnosis. While this technically qualifies as an internal motivation, it is unhealthy and could be too little too late. Don't get me wrong, it's never too late to start a fitness program, as they are beneficial at all ages and stages of life, but the sooner, the better. What matters more is that it comes from the right type of internal motivation such as pursuing happiness, enjoyment, and satisfaction.[49]

It's very important to distinguish the difference between understanding something is good for you and having internal motivation to actually go complete that something. The key word here is *understanding*. It's not enough to just understand how you think you should get to your goals or what things to avoid that could prevent you from reaching them. Deeper than the desire, it means becoming educated on a topic if you ever want to accomplish a goal. I think this is where most people fall short. Internal motivation can keep a fire lit underneath you to learn about a topic or seek out the right help to reach your goals safely, but you also have to connect that desire to knowledge. In other words, the goal itself isn't enough on its own— you need to delve deeper into a topic and learn everything you can.

Everybody knows that an apple is healthier than a candy bar, but what they may not know is that by completely restricting the candy bar from their diet cold turkey, they may cause further cravings for the candy bar. So if your goal was to eat fewer candy bars by ridding your house of all things candy and sweets, you may be doing a disservice to your goals by restricting too much and then binging later on. You will feel shame or disappointment and may ultimately give up on your goal. If your goal was to get in better physical shape but you don't seek out the help of the proper professional, you will most likely end up doing a thirty or ninety-day challenge and, even if you complete it find yourself falling back out of shape or getting injured in the process within six months. Again, it wouldn't be enough to just

---

49   Gemma Maria Gea-García, Noelia González-Gálvez, Alejandro Espeso-García, Pablo J. Marcos-Pardo, Francisco Tomás González-Fernández, Luis Manuel Martínez-Aranda, "Relationship Between the Practice of Physical Activity and Physical Fitness in Physical Education Students: The Integrated Regulation As a Mediating Variable," *Frontiers in Psychology* 11 (2020): 1910, https://doi.org/10.3389/fpsyg.2020.01910.

find a professional. You would have to learn more about the industry to find a professional that fits your needs.

Ultimately, that's why those people showed up for my talk … they wanted to learn. They were already motivated to be healthy but recognized they needed to grow their knowledge. But an essential part of learning is knowing the right questions to ask. Now, it's one thing to motivate a group of strangers in a room who came to hear you of their own free will seeking that knowledge. It's a whole other thing to motivate those you are closest to.

## Motivating Your Loved Ones

So maybe you're reading this and saying to yourself, "Yeah, but how can I motivate someone if it's in their best interest? Is *all* external motivation ineffective? Or can external motivation be turned into internal motivation?" Typically, these questions come up with loved ones, not the stranger you pass by in the grocery store.

In my experience, the closer you are to the person, the harder it may be to get your message across, especially with a potentially sensitive topic like fitness. Whether someone is your spouse, partner, sibling, or best friend, you might have a past history of commenting on their appearance or directing their attention toward certain habits. If these previous interactions went well, helping them find internal motivation may be easy. But if those times did not go well, then this might be a real uphill battle.

> Sometimes they won't listen to you *because* you are too close.

It's logical to think that as a loved one, the other person should just listen to you, but many times, it's the opposite. Sometimes they won't listen to you *because* you are too close, and because you know them so well, you might even forget that they need to be persuaded and introduced to new ideas in their own specific ways. I've seen this in my own family.

Now, it's important to understand that my father, Bill, also has a very strict dietary routine and his own very unique take on health. What I mean is that every day for breakfast he has a pork chop with applesauce, then for his first lunch he eats a turkey burger with a sweet potato, the second lunch a salad of some kind, and dinner is a coin flip between Italian or Chinese, then a snack at night. But whether it ends up being Italian or Chinese for dinner, he gets the same dishes every time.

I can remember this type of behavior all the way back to when I was a kid. After my Little League baseball games, we would go to the diner by our old house where he would order, "Diet Coke with no ice and three pieces of lemon" every time. Yes, every time—and yes, exactly three pieces of lemon. Nowadays, he drinks mostly water but will have a Diet Coke once a day, still with no ice. The lemon became less important, but the "no ice" request has stuck around because he says the melting ice waters down the taste of the Diet Coke.

When even something as simple as that gets stuck in somebody's head, it will keep them from changing forever. It's just a thought he had once when having Diet Coke, and right then he decided, "From now on, this is how I will enjoy soda." Hot day? Doesn't matter, no ice. Large versus small size? That also doesn't matter, no ice. The point is he is a very rigid man. Once he gets his mind stuck on something, it will forever need to be that way, and I think that's a pretty common behavior across the entire human species.

So who should understand that more than his wife of twenty years, Jeana? She holds a PhD in psychology from UCLA and has studied human psychology and behavior change for five decades. But it almost seems all of that knowledge and experience is nullified with my father, so I think it's fair to say that it's normal for the average person to struggle with communicating with a loved one.

Father's Day two weeks after my dad's seventy-third birthday provided a solid example of how this played out. After we finished some delicious pork chops that my father had prepared for all of us, we sat around talking. Jeana looked at me with a very serious and concerned look on her face and said, "Your dad's too skinny. He's lost ten pounds in the last few months. Tell him to eat more."

My dad chimed in, "I eat the same as I've always eaten. I just burn between 2,500 and 3,000 calories a day."

Jeana continued, "I keep telling him to eat more. It's not healthy for him to be losing weight at this rate! When I first met him [over twenty years ago], he was two hundred pounds, and a few years ago, he was perfect at 175. Now he's 153, and I'm nervous something's wrong."

"Jeana, I'm eating plenty," he responded. "I do my five meals a day. There's not much more I can eat."

As they continued, I found out that at his doctor's office five months before, he had weighed 163 pounds with clothes on in the middle of the day. Then, when he weighed himself on his home scale, he was 153 in the morning without clothes, and then 157 with clothes later in the day. He'd had blood work done recently and a full workup, and all else seemed normal. Now, it's also important to note that Jeana has always wanted my father to gain more muscle, so for as long as I can remember, she's been pushing him to exercise more and therefore pushing *me* to teach him exercises. But as a son to a father, communication is very different, so it has been an uphill battle for me too.

I had gotten him a Fitbit for his birthday two years before. He hated it at first but wears it religiously now, which—again—is very fitting to his personality. Bill isn't one to exercise with weights, but he enjoys his morning floor band exercise routine and his daily walk. Now as much as I've talked about progressive overload and the need to change your fitness program every four to eight weeks, he's heard the concept ten times over but has never adopted the principle himself. So step one was to make him aware of his movement in a way that a regimented man would take to the idea.

A tracking device was perfect: it would give him a way to quantify his daily activity and track it more accurately. Now again, tracking devices (like weight scales) can be off, even upward of 10–20 percent, but if you use the same one daily, you will be able to see if the numbers go up or down, regardless of whether they are originally off. Needless to say, my external motivation gesture turned into an internal motivation for my father to attain his specific goals we set with him on the Fitbit.

With all that said, Jeana continued by asking me, "Did you notice he has lost more weight?"

Before I could even respond, my dad said, "When I saw I had lost weight, I tried this shirt on because it didn't fit well before, and now it fits great."

For the past few years, this was his thing. He loved to tell you how skinny he was. He would stand up tall, tap his stomach, and say, "Look at how skinny I am. I'm in the best shape of my life." Then he would proceed to flex his elbow and make a tight bicep. "Feel how solid my arms are. Not bad for a seventy-year-old man, huh?"

So part of what Jeana was missing was that my father *liked* the idea that he was skinny and for her to perceive him as too skinny was almost the ultimate compliment. Every time she would say, "Bill, you're too skinny," he would hear, "Bill, you look great," even if she literally followed up her statement with how it looks unhealthy or less attractive. He even wore a shirt that used to be too small for him to see if I would notice the difference. That is not a sign of a man who is willing to gain weight or even who wouldn't want to lose even more weight. So if someone as knowledgeable about human psychology as Jeana could miss this point of view, then it's safe to assume the average person could miss these types of cues with their loved ones.

Did you notice what else she did incorrectly?

She demanded for him to *gain* weight, embarrassing him by passively saying he doesn't look good in front of his own son, which will only cause him to block out what she's saying and strengthen his own point of view. When we speak from only our own point of view without consideration of our loved one's viewpoint, we may unintentionally put up a wall rather than motivate them.

Also, she gave him no goal, which is essential for motivation. He's a regimented guy who likes structure, so if you tell him his current structure is wrong, he will only convince himself *you're* wrong because you didn't provide any replacement structure or stepping stones to a new structure.

You may have noticed she also discussed how he *used* to look and at what weight she liked him best. Jeana meant it to be motivating, but she was operating under the false illusion that he would want to be the weight *she* found the most appealing and not the weight *he* enjoyed the most.

Finally, she tried to force him into a habit change through only external motivation. Bill needed internal motivation to make these major lifestyle changes, to alter the way he sees his body, and how he views his health standards. This is why it's too simple to just think somebody should be motivated because a loved one tells them to change—it *has* to come from within.

# Motivation for Tomorrow

Now, maybe you're like the nurse and other medical professionals who came to my talk, hungry for knowledge borne out of an internal motivation. The question I have for you is "What are you going to do with that motivation? How are you going to apply this knowledge tomorrow to make changes in your health and fitness journey?"

Or maybe you're being externally motivated by a friend who recommended this book to you. If so, they obviously understood how to communicate the proper way to spark a little fire in you because if you've made it this far, then it must have generated at least some internal motivation for you to fan the flames and hopefully turn into a full-blown raging fire. So if that's your situation, well, I have the exact same questions for you too: "What will you do with that motivation, and how will you apply this knowledge tomorrow?"

My hope, of course, is that you will choose to be an agent of change for the fitness industry by identifying the right goals and finding the right FP to help you achieve those goals. Furthermore, I hope this book will be your guide to finding that right professional, which we'll talk about in the next chapter. After that, I'm hoping you pass on that knowledge to others, creating the snowball effect that I believe will lead to lasting change in this industry.

So when you recommend this book to other people, some may read it and love it while others just look at the cover and throw it back. Some may even shut down the conversation about the book before you can get another word in. I think this has little to do with the book itself (I won't give myself that much credit), but more to do with how you framed and communicated the message, their current frame of mind, and your relationship to them. If you are their mentor, they will read the book, like I did when *How to Eat, Move, and Be Healthy* was recommended to me because I knew Dr. Thomas was knowledgeable in subjects that interested me. If you are a friend who has gone through a similar journey, your friend may listen to you because of the respect they have for your accomplishments. No matter what, I think it's important as we near the end of our discussion to emphasize that the conversation doesn't stop here and that what's more important is how you apply your newfound motivation and knowledge tomorrow.

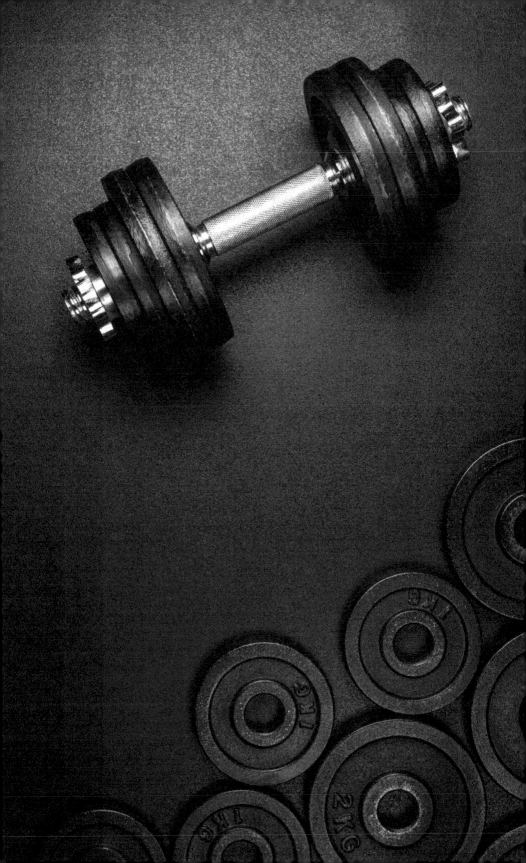

CHAPTER 10

# Finding Your New Gym, Workouts, and Fitness Professional

*Culture is the arts elevated to a set of beliefs.*
—THOMAS WOLFE

Waiting for a call back from any job interview can be nerve-racking. It was the end of summer after I had completed undergraduate school, and I had applied to work as a personal trainer for the top two fitness companies in New York. After being called in and completing interviews at both clubs, it was a waiting game. Two weeks after my interview, I was driving to a birthday dinner my family was having for me at our favorite Italian restaurant when my phone rang. It was the best birthday present to find out that I had received the job and would be starting the next week.

The next few weeks would teach me more about the industry itself than any book, DVD/video collection, mentor, or even college class ever could. On day one, I received one light blue shirt with the name of the company and the word "trainer" on the back. It's important to note that all the "established" trainers in the company received black shirts—and more than just one. My personal training manager at the time had told me that I would be learning the company's assessment process before I was allowed to take on any clients. However, in the meantime, I would "walk the floor," cleaning up and organizing the gym floor while handing out towels to members and building rapport with them.

Over the next month, I would have at least four floor shifts a week with hours ranging from 5:00 to 9:00 a.m. and 5:00 to 9:00 p.m. To become a successful personal trainer in today's world, passing online exams can be easy, getting a job at the local gym can be easy, even getting clients can be easy, but working a closing shift followed by a morning floor shift for months while only making $8/hour is never easy. So whether it was the company's intention or not, this type of introduction creates a high turnover rate. You will either quit in the first few months or you'll develop a hunger to "get off the floor" and start training.

But here's the problem. The only way to get off the floor is to become a full-time trainer, and the only way to become a full-time trainer is to hit a certain number of completed training sessions each month. Thus, this hunger, like a starved beast in a cage, turns you into a sales monster. Once the personal training manager thinks you have learned their assessment well enough, they will give you the green light to find clients. You are then released from your restraints and now see all members as future paying clients. You are a free sales lion now, and nobody can tame you, not even your own morals. The need to get off the floor begins to supersede your desire to help clients because it becomes more important to wear the black shirt and work the floor shifts if you want to become full time and apply for health and financial benefits.

Three months after my first day, and two months after I had been cleared to take on clients, I managed to muster up … one client. She was a nineteen-year-old girl who had her father pay for one package of sessions because she thought I was cute. So naturally, I began to contemplate if fitness was really the path for me. I was drained of all excitement to help the world, to gain more knowledge, and to lead a change effort in the industry. In place of that happiness, I was just filled with feelings of hopelessness, confusion, and lack of passion.

Explaining the science of exercise and the idea that results take a long time to build did not seem to be working well for me. My father, who had spent over forty years in sales at the time, would constantly give me advice and pep talks to keep me going, but to no avail. The morning of my fourth month, I woke up and said to myself, "If I don't make it this month, I'm quitting the fitness industry and going to find a career in real estate" (another passion of mine). I made it a mantra on my drive to work every day to repeat, "I'm going to sell at least two clients today" while I listened to audiobooks on sales, including everything and anything, from the old-school *The Psychology of Selling* by Brian Tracy to new age *Sell or Be Sold* by Grant Cardone.

I spoke to everybody who walked onto the floor. If you were a member, you got a towel whether you wanted one or not. I would interject myself into someone's workout and offer up unsolicited corrections and alternatives. If you had been there, you couldn't leave the gym without getting either a "Hi" or "Bye"—or both—from me. I was using lines like, "Sure, I can show you a quick exercise for your abs … but I can also give you a fish and you can eat for a day, or I can teach you how to fish and you can eat forever. Come use your free assessment with me, and I'll make sure you can train properly for the rest of your life!"

I booked and sold nineteen clients that month, breaking that club location's record. I was now off the floor and training clients. Some at 5:00 a.m., some at 10:00 a.m., some at 2:00 p.m., and even some at 9:00 p.m. Within the next two years, I would jump from what was considered Level 1 to one of the top levels in the club. I was full time, sporting the coveted black shirt every day. I made my own schedule, was hitting club bonuses, and … I was miserable. Personal training had become a sales and entertainment game. I was no longer on a mission to change lives; I was on a mission to hit bonuses and make more money by training more people.

While this was a top global fitness company, their business model showed they were clearly all about revenue first. So the more people you trained, the more money they made. This created a cycle of "sell more because you're still not good enough." When personal training is a third of the total company's revenue, it's important to keep training more and more clients. If you want a vacation—or even a few days off—another trainer must train your clients because if your numbers begin to fall, you would be punished, whether financially (smaller bonus) or scolded in the office with clear doors for all your coworkers to see. If you're home sick with the flu, who is covering your sessions? If nobody, they would pull the sessions anyway, and it was your job to make up those sessions at a later date "off the books" because that client still needed to get their usual number of sessions in that next week as well, regardless of your personal circumstances.

I used to go home exhausted and say to myself, "This is no way to help people. I can't be giving up my values—or my own health—just to make money. There has to be a better way."

So just before the two-year mark, I left the company and opened my business. I knew something new needed to emerge, and I was going to create it. Within five years, I learned I couldn't make this change alone.

I say all this to point out that, as an insider of the industry who loves fitness as much as I do who almost lost that love, I can completely understand how easy it could be for a member of the public to lose interest and burn out. And since the industry isn't going to change today—or even tomorrow—and it certainly won't change all at once, I think we have to talk about how you can work within the current system to find the "right fit" for which gym to choose and what to look for in a fitness professional.

## Selecting the Right Gym/Center

Since the age of sixteen, I have been a member of different gyms: LA Fitness, Gold's, Synergy, Lifetime, Equinox, small local gyms, even boxing and mixed martial arts (MMA) gyms. They were all so different yet also very similar. The equipment all looked the same, the gym floors always looked familiar, but some were cleaner than others, some had more qualified trainers than others. Size always seemed to make a difference in what equipment was there, but they always felt equally packed regardless of their square footage. It was always amazing to me to walk through a front door of a gym and be greeted by name when you knew they had thousands of members, but the clients that came to see me hated that and preferred the small studio experience.

Certain gyms loved to blast music throughout the day, so loud that you couldn't even hear your own music through your headphones while other gyms wouldn't play music at all and if you took your headphones out, it was the most demotivating experience you can imagine. But to offset that lack of quality, the "music-less" gyms would have equipment or their walls bright colors like orange, red, or yellow. Still other gyms wouldn't dare to do something they considered cheap or tacky and went with more of an upscale feel with a marble front desk and state-of-the-art equipment.

Then came my favorite difference. There was always a range across the gym spectrum of *community*. You could make an argument that the gyms who knew your first name and had spoken to you behind a marble desk were building community through brand marketing, but that's not what I'm talking about. I'm talking about the sense of community that emerges among the community of members themselves. Some of the smallest gyms, ones with the worst training systems and cheapest equipment, had the strongest sense of community while some of the gyms with large cafés, seating areas, monthly events, and so on had the worst member-to-member connection.

> You need to find the right trainer and the right community that will help spur you on to accomplish your goals.

In the last chapter, you may have begun to explore the reasons why you want to get into fitness today or even which gym in your local area seems to be the right fit. Now I want you to dive deeper and really think about all the attributes that go into making a gym your second home. Gym memberships are far from cheap, and to get your money's worth, you need to find the right one. Then you need to find the right trainer and the right community that will help spur you on to accomplish your goals. This will directly correlate to the amount of time you spend at the gym, the number of years you belong to the gym, the friends you will make, the results you will achieve, and your overall view of fitness.

# Selecting the Right Professional

When it comes to selecting the right trainer/FP/EP, I think it simplifies everything if you think of exercise as a sport. If you wanted to play baseball, even just recreationally, you would need to learn how. You can't just show up to the field day one of the league with some dusty old mitt you found in your attic, a borrowed wooden bat, and no knowledge of how to play the game and expect to be able to play well. Sure, you may catch a ball on pure instinct. From the MLB games you've watched, you may understand what a swing should look like and how to run the bases, but you'll strike out too many times to even make it to first base. All around, it would be a rough day.

If you were serious about getting better or learning the game, what would you do next? You can't go to the batting cages and practice yet, because maybe you don't understand the mechanics of a swing. So just like personal training, you don't need to understand anatomy and biomechanics or physiology and biotensegrity[50] to make contact with the ball, but you do need a good coach who understands the science behind swing mechanics. The coach would teach you how not only to make contact, but what pitches to swing at and which to avoid. You would also learn how to run the bases, catch a ball properly, what equipment you should or should not use, the rules of the game, the history of the game, and much more.

The point is, you could painfully learn baseball by yourself over a decade, striking out at every game until you get a hit, using an old glove until your hand hurts trying to catch a ball, and losing the passion for the game before it even starts, or you could hire a coach and grow your game exponentially in a much shorter period of time.

---

50   Graham Scarr, *Biotensegrity: The Structural Basis of Life*, 2nd ed. (Pencaitland, Scotland: Handspring Pub Ltd., 2019).

Experts, coaches, and mentors teach you in a few hours what it took them decades to learn. It's why we put our kids in organized sports with coaches. It's why when you start out in fitness, you need an educated coach, ideally an exercise physiologist, to coach you through the science behind the right exercise for you. Like coaches, there are a wide variety to choose from.

There are a lot of trainers in the world who really *do* want to help people. They want to change people's lives and they are not in it for the money, but far too many of them didn't learn the science behind not only the exercises they are teaching their clients, but the science of exercise as a whole.

The key is finding the right fitness professional. Even if they are a virtual or at-home personal trainer, it matters what gym companies they have worked for in the past, because those work cultures will shape the perspective the trainer has. If they started in a gym whose ideals are totally different from your goals, then that trainer may not be right for you. Remember, everything is interconnected. The trainer is a product of their education and gym history, the physical therapist is impacted by the network they surround themselves with, including the exercise physiologists, and the medical community is integrally linked to the results you see from your gym and fitness professional.

## Selecting the Right Plan/Program

Picking the right fitness professional really goes hand in hand with what kind of program you need. But no matter what, a good rule of thumb is looking at whether their focus is on helping you with gradual progress while preventing injury or whether they are just "quick fixers" roping you in with promises of fast results through more reps, more intensity.

Instead, a true trainer/FP/EP should be asking you, "How do you want to feel?" From there, if they have your best interest in mind, they can work with you on how your program should "feel" by picking how many days a week you work out, how long you exercise, what exercise means to *you*, where you exercise, and what your micro and macro goals are. As we discussed before, your new goals can be as simple as "I want to be able to walk into the house holding all the groceries in one trip" or "I want to play with my kids outside until they're tired." In this case, the quick-fix ten-minute ab workout a trainer/program is trying to push on you may not be appropriate for your lifestyle or goal.

If endurance is your target, your trainer should be utilizing a program that may need to include more stair work and fewer bicep curls, targeting the same muscles you'll be using carrying those groceries or playing with your kids. You may begin to see a deadlift (lifting weight off the floor) as an exercise you *want* to do when it was previously your least favorite exercise.

With the right trainer who is focused on your goals, fitness takes on a new meaning now because it's defined by your needs, not someone else's idea of what it should be. But the irony is that the "redefining" really just brings the original definition of fitness back to the light. As you search for your trainer, I want you to try to reimagine everything you once knew or associated with fitness and the exercise industry based not on what will build a six-pack but will build a better future for you.

## Questions for Finding Answers

Obviously, I can't sit down with each of you to get to know you and your needs and then pinpoint the perfect gym or trainer for you, as much as I'd love to. But as I've hinted at previously, I think the best way to find the right answers for you is knowing the right questions to ask. So here are some things you need to be asking at every stage of your fitness journey.

## MOTIVATION AND FINDING A GYM

1. Am I internally motivated to engage in a program right now? If not, why not? What is standing in my way, and how can I overcome those obstacles?

2. Do I want a boutique experience, a place where I can build a relationship with other regular members? Do I want a local "mom and pop" shop to support?

3. Do I want a place where everyone knows my name—or do I want a place where people will leave me the heck alone so I can have some "me" time?

4. Do I travel a lot and need a membership at a chain gym I can find pretty much anywhere so that I can't make the excuse of not working out when I'm on the road?

5. Do other members look like me or represent the results I am looking to achieve? Are there programs there that actually interest me or just the fad workout of the year? (for example, do you want an indoor track to use? Or a kickboxing class? Or a pool? Or even a rock-climbing wall? Or are you perfectly happy with a basic set of dumbbells, treadmill, and bench?)

6. Do I want to work out one-on-one with somebody? In an intimate group? Or do I prefer large group classes?

## QUESTIONS TO ASK AT THE GYM

The previous set of questions deals more with the general vibe of the gym, but it's also important to know questions you can ask the gym personnel before you make a commitment.

1.  Which trainers here have a degree in exercise science or a related field? (Note: physiology is a popular degree for some reason, but is not directly related to fitness/exercise, in contrast to exercise physiology.)

2.  Do you have anyone on your staff who specializes in my need for _____? (for example, corrective exercise, injury prevention, improving daily movement, weight loss, etc.) Do they have specialty certifications?

3.  What is the trainer's educational background and require-ments? Do they have training/working knowledge in an allied field such as physical therapy or any medical training? Do you have certified exercise physiologists?

4.  Who has the highest reviews in the gym from clients with similar goals to mine and why? (Note: "why" being the most important question because with the knowledge learned from this book, you should be able to decide if their answer is what you were hoping to hear.)

5.  What is the goal for me at the end of each workout?

This last question is intended directly for the potential trainer you are "interviewing." If they respond that it is "to be sweaty or tired," then it's my view that is the wrong trainer/gym for you. You need to see if they have the outdated "no pain, no gain" mentality. The goal *should* be to feel accomplished, stronger, healthier, and progressing without injury. If you are tired or sweaty as a result, that is fine, and it may be part of the process, but sweat and exhaustion are not markers of a good workout in and of themselves.

## QUESTIONS TO ASK YOURSELF AT THE GYM

1. Does the trainer recommended to me have a personality that I will respond positively and happily to?

2. Is the trainer or program given to me setting realistic guidelines that I would actually be able to follow?

3. After your first workout: Do I feel strong, empowered, and motivated for more, or do I just feel overly exhausted and drenched in sweat?

## RED FLAGS

Finally, I want to leave you with what I would consider some "red flags" for when you may need to leave a gym—or never join it to begin with. These are the sort of things that, if you know what to look for, can end up saving you time, money, energy, and possibly save you from injury:

1. Many trainers like training clients in the way that they themselves like to work out or look. What works for them may not work for you, though. So if the trainer looks like a magazine cover and seems to think you need to look just like them, it may be best to find another. In other words, are they taking your unique interests and abilities into consideration, or are they just trying to turn you into a clone of themselves?

2. It's a huge red flag if you feel like you are being pushed into buying sessions or a membership before the trainer or

sales staff has a chance to really evaluate and/or get to know you. Why would you join their couch to 5K in thirty days program if you don't care about running a 5K and you're just looking to feel better?

3. A lack of professional attire should set off another red flag. A tank top or a sleeveless shirt is not conducive to a professional environment. At minimum, a short-sleeved collared shirt and full-length pants (workout pants are okay) should be expected.

4. "Cleanliness is next to godliness." The gym is dirtier than it looks, so if it *looks* dirty, you may not even want to touch the door on the way out.

5. Look at the gym's marketing. What do you see on the pictures on their walls, advertisements, and signs? If they don't look relatable, it may be best to try somewhere else. Don't just try to fit into the current fitness mold because it will be changing soon, and you should strive to be ahead of the curve.

## QUESTIONS FOR STARTING AN ONLINE OR VIRTUAL PROGRAM

Now, I'm aware not everyone lives in an area with many gym choices. Maybe you have no choices. Or even if you do, your lifestyle or budget may not accommodate you jumping right into a membership or using a fitness professional right off the bat. That's okay. Don't wait to start your fitness journey until all these conditions are perfect. If you have to do an online or virtual program, you can still make wise choices.

1. What are my goals, and will this program help me accomplish them? If so, how specifically?

2. How can the instructor really tailor the program to my unique needs if it's prerecorded or working with hundreds of people at once? Is it time-driven, or is there any focus on good form?

3. Do the trainers and assistants in the videos look like what I am trying to achieve?

4. Does the program include any exercises or conversation about injury prevention? Does the program offer modifications if an exercise can't be completed because of my condition?

5. Is this program well-organized/logical/systematic, or does it seem like random exercises placed together and paced at a level that will just make me sweaty?

6. Does this program take into consideration things like my age or exercise interests? Are there options for me to modify it based on my BMI, age, medical history, etc.?

Don't get me wrong—there is no "perfect" solution where all of your concerns will be addressed. One day, I hope we get there, but we're just not there yet. At least with these questions, you can prioritize what is most important for you and, frankly, you can help drive change in the industry. If a gym is willing to listen to your goals, your concerns, they may well be worth sticking with even if they don't have everything you're looking for.

Most of today's personal trainers may ask you general questions about your goals, but there's a good chance they assume

> **It's more important to find the person who will listen to your true goals that go deeper, the ones based in feeling better and moving better.**

it's aesthetics and weight loss. It's more important to find the person who will listen to your true goals that go deeper, the ones based in feeling better and moving better. You can change those assumptions based on your questions and choices. Those choices can cause a ripple effect in the industry that will lead to lasting change that can make our world a better, healthier, less-injured place.

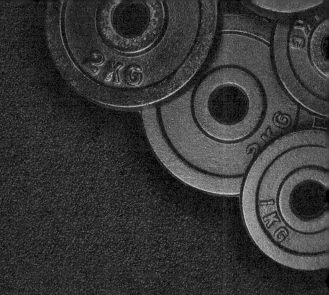

CONCLUSION:

# Post-Workout

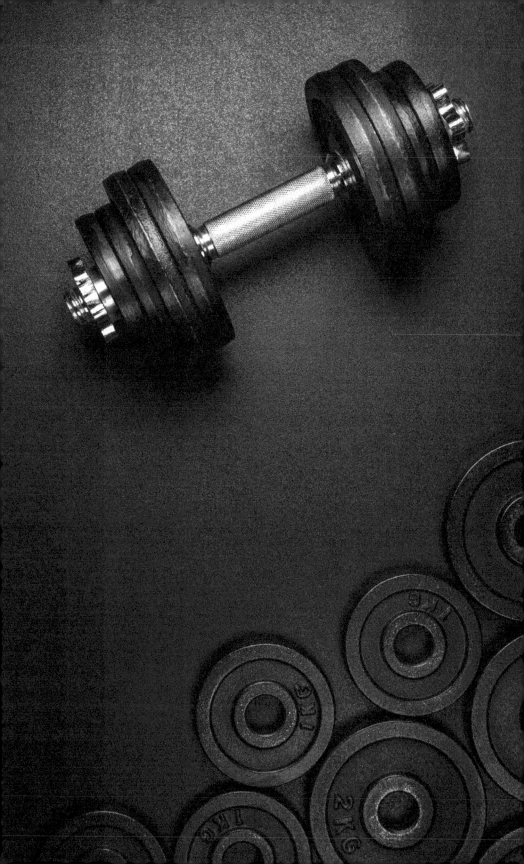

# What You Need to Do Now

*It's never too late to become who you want to be. I hope*
*you live a life that you're proud of, and if you find that*
*you're not, I hope you have the strength to start over.*
—F. SCOTT FITZGERALD

When I was eight years old, my parents enrolled me in a soccer league. And just like with my T-ball league and my tennis league, my father volunteered to be the coach or the assistant coach of our team. As I mentioned earlier, my father spent decades in sales, so he didn't have much time for a professional career as a soccer player. Instead, he spent countless hours watching DVDs on soccer and reading articles on drills to do with kids and a few books on coaching. All this effort to make sure that his son learned the proper way to play the game.

To make a long story short, the results can be summed up in his two favorite lines: "Just boot the ball" and "Shoot as much as possible." His logic here was "If the ball is on their side of the field, they can't score." Needless to say, my soccer career didn't last very long. The intention my father had to be by my side to encourage me and help me grow was something very few sons get to feel, but the lack of practical knowledge in the sport led to the ultimate failure in the methodology. Good intentions, but not so good execution.

## FITNESS PROFESSIONALS/GENERAL PUBLIC

Perspective shift from aesthetics to injury prevention/better movement.

## FITNESS PROFESSIONALS/MEDICAL AND ALLIED MEDICAL COMMUNITY

Develop means for better communication/collaboration between FPs and the medical community.

## FITNESS PROFESSIONALS/GYM OWNERS

Raise the bar of knowledge and skills for FPs to better address the needs present in the public.

## GENERAL PUBLIC

Demand more holistic-focused programs and higher level of education for professionals.

And that's how I see the current state of the fitness industry: good intentions, but not so good execution. And while I know it's unrealistic to think one person can change things all alone, I'm hopeful we can improve the industry if each of us will commit to execute our part, no matter where you are in the industry:

Once we can each take ownership of our part of change, then change can truly start to happen. This means not only having a more holistic view of health and fitness as individuals, but also as a society and industry. When that happens, we can make a real difference.

I've told stories of both my parents' roles in how I became so interested in what's wrong with all our current healthcare and preventative wellness systems. I never finished the Father's Day story from chapter nine because the end can sum up the entire structural problem in the fitness industry, which is what I want to leave you with.

As you might remember, my stepmother, Jeana, was trying to motivate my father based on her view of what was good for him rather than looking from his point of view. After we started reframing how Jeana communicates to my father, we set some next steps for him to begin a new view on his health and wellness by discussing his fitness habits.

I said, "Dad, a reason you may be seeing the weight loss you're so proud of is if you have osteoporosis. I remember you mentioned having some in your hip a few years back, but it can manifest in other areas of the body as well. I know we've talked for years about adding external weights to your morning fitness routine, but have you tried anything new or looked into changing up the exercises?"

He responded in the most American view of healthcare I could ever cite: "What do you mean?" He was genuinely confused and continued, "I do the morning exercises every morning. I can't change them. Everything else hurts my back. I walk every day, I do the exercises the PT gave me [years ago], and I take my calcium and other vitamins for strong bones."

See the problems here? Pills for "quick-fix" stronger bones, no follow-up on an exercise program from a physical therapist years before, no seeking an exercise professional's help (even though his son is one), the certainty he is already doing everything possible, and the false confidence that he mistakenly put in the current healthcare system. He was seventy-three, taking upward of fifty pills a day and suffering from chronic, crippling back pain and unhealthy, unexplained weight loss. He was using exercises designed for one goal (back pain) created years ago with no teaching of how he can progress the program for his current state and no current supervision in terms of his health and lifestyle, yet he had convinced himself he was the pillar of health for his age. The bar we have set for healthcare and preventative wellness is extremely low, the current system we use is terribly broken, and the mindset of

> The current system we use is terribly broken, and the mindset of the average American is flawed.

the average American is flawed at the expense of their own quality of life and longevity.

Yes, we have a long way to go as a fitness industry and even further to go as an allied medical/wellness community. Again, this ranges on the spectrum of preventative wellness (fitness, nutrition, and so on) to the conventional medical practice of being treated after you're already sick or injured. Insurance companies, hospital systems, and allied medical communities will play a large role in this change in the years to come, but it's *you* and the general public who will be the greatest agents of change. The demand for better fitness, better networking, and a new view of healthcare will push each industry to change and come together.

Even the shift of the internal motivators from "How can I lose weight now?" to "How can I improve my movement and quality of life long term?" will be an ongoing battle for most people. After all, we have an image-centric culture and are constantly comparing ourselves to others, whether celebrities or our friends on social media posting idyllic "beach body" pics. Know that this struggle is okay and just part of the natural process of change. You must give yourself permission to not be perfect every day and give yourself the freedom to not be on a strict exercise regimen or try to look like someone else. Just like a quality fitness program, your own personal beliefs take a long time to produce the results that you would like to see today. It is all a process.

In the meantime, I really hope this book serves to be the first of not just small stepping stones, but giant leaps in these changes happening. I myself have had to come to terms with the idea that this industry and medical community change may not happen in my lifetime. But change won't happen if we don't talk about it, so you can help continue the conversation by asking the questions from the last chapter and bringing up some—or all—of these ideas with others in your community.

In light of that reality, we have to focus on what we can control *today*. That is your own view and actions toward fitness, how deeply you understand the seemingly confusing world of exercise, and how well you navigate it. Once we understand the world around us, we can begin to make change. If you understand that the current field of exercise is pushing quick fixes, it becomes your responsibility to seek out a better option. It is the fault of the industry for pushing these methods, but once you are exposed to the truth, your personal responsibility for bettering yourself falls on you and your choices.

> We have to focus on what we can control *today*.

Maybe you're reading this because you don't struggle with starting to exercise, but maybe it's become an obsession for you. Fitness disorders/disordered fitness are real things, so basing how much you eat in a day on how much you exercise is disordered. You also have to fight the feeling of shame or self-loathing that you may get if a day or even a few days go by without exercising. The same can be said if you feel the need to exercise even when you're injured because you have a deep-seated belief that exercising is the only way to be healthy.

As someone who's been around the fitness industry my entire life, I want you to know it's not your fault if these ideas have constantly bombarded you every day throughout your entire life. Hopefully, you now have the tools to let go of those negative ideas, shift your perspective, and create a healthier relationship with fitness.

I know that some of what I propose throughout the book is unconventional and even controversial in today's climate. But I'd be remiss to not share what I've learned both from firsthand experience and the latest research in fitness and exercise. So regardless of who you are or where you are on the spectrum of fitness, you now have the knowledge to go out into the world, see the system's imperfections, change your belief system, help those around you, and personally choose the right exercise professional to help you, the right gym culture to immerse yourself in, and the ability to create realistic goals based on the quality of your longevity.

You have a choice before you. I can't make you go to the gym, put the extra effort in to find the right professional, or even change your current fitness programs and habits. So the question is what *you* will do with this knowledge: Will you apply it? Or put down this book and move on, business as usual? If you do nothing and continue to practice "unprotected sets" in our aesthetics-obsessed, quick-fix culture, experience has taught me that your chance of injury is high, which could ultimately cause you to become disillusioned and give up the idea of fitness for yourself or passively allow others to get injured or give up.

Instead, I'd encourage you to do something with this knowledge. Take action and start simple—you don't have to do everything at once. Sit down and figure out your macro goal, and work backward from there. Take your time and make sure you use the guidelines learned throughout this book to make more informed choices. Talk to your doctor or PT or trainer about what you've learned.

But I'd also encourage you to look beyond yourself and your needs, as important as those things are. Think about who else you know needs to hear this message: a friend, a family member, your doctor? Who else needs to read this because it could change their life?

I think back to that first day of class when Dr. Jackson asked about the number of reps and sets for building muscle mass. If she'd never shared that information with me, I might still be stuck in the old way of thinking "more is better" and "no pain, no gain." Not only did that change my own life and the way that I pursue fitness, but it changed the way I help others every day. Now think about what a difference it could make not just for you, but for your friends and loved ones—and then the country—if we can start to implement these small changes for a healthier society. How many lives could be saved? How many more of life's moments could we enjoy instead of being hindered by pain?

We all have to do our part and take the small steps that will lead to giant leaps in fitness and health. When you make the choice to take those small steps, you will be playing your part in changing the fitness industry and building a world that practices "safe sets."

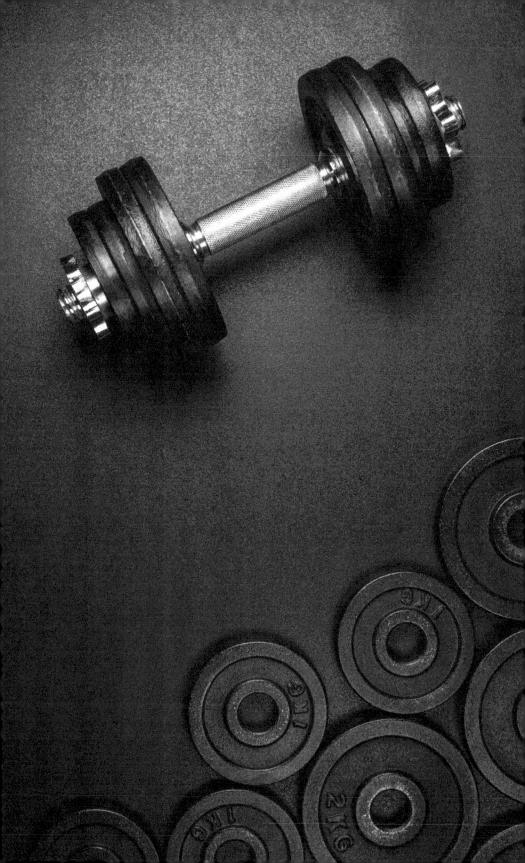

# Glossary

**Allied Health Community**—Large scope of different types of professionals and specialists working with patients with specific health needs, such as physical therapists, occupational therapists, chiropractors, and registered dieticians, among others.

**Chiropractor (chiro)**—Specialist who focuses on the musculoskeletal system in their patients.

**Corrective Exercise Specialist (CES)**—Certified fitness professional who specializes in exercise and fitness practices with the intention of correcting movement and reducing the risk of injury.

**Exercise/Injury (E/I) Cycle**—A "hamster wheel" cycle that includes injury/pain, medical care, physical therapy, and exercise programs.

**Exercise Physiologist (EP)**—In the context of this book, the highest level of fitness professional who holds a bachelor's degree (or even a master's) in exercise physiology and is certified through a reputable organization such as ACSM (American College of Sports Medicine) or NASM (National Academy of Sports Medicine), along with other specialty certifications.

**Fascia**—Thin tissue that encases and connects every part of your body, including organs, muscles, bones, nerves, and blood vessels.

**Fitness Professional (FP)**—Commonly used as a blanket term for anyone working in the fitness industry. In the context of this book, I use it to refer to someone who focuses on coaching an individual by knowing them on a personal level, including understanding their unique health goals and needs and how they should align with their fitness plan while also considering their mental and social health.

**Functional Exercises**—Exercises designed to train the body for activities you might do in your day-to-day life, like standing from a seated position or reaching for a glass on the top shelf.

**Health Community/Health Professional**—Medical doctors and nurses.

**Holistic**—Having a 360-degree view of an individual, understanding someone beyond their external aesthetics and being able to see them inside and out, what's going on in their mind, spirit, and body.

**Occupational Therapist (OT)**—Specialist who focuses more on helping patients with being able to handle everyday living skills, functional movement, balance, and coordination.

**Personal Trainer**—In the context of this book, the most common worker in the fitness industry, ranging from gym trainer working the floor, exercise class leader, or even HIIT instructor. May range from someone working part time or full time, various levels of education and certification, including no formal education or just an online certification. Often focuses purely on aesthetics, general weight loss, or represents a specific workout program.

**Physical Therapist (PT)**—Includes specialists in both rehabilitation therapy (after surgery) or prehabilitation therapy (before surgery), often helping patients recuperate or regain strength and movement following an injury or surgery.

**Prehabilitation (prehab)**—Exercises and fitness practices designed to improve a patient's health before surgery under the direction of an EP. Includes corrective exercises prescribed and utilized to lower the risk of injury before a person begins training, as identified in an evaluation.

**Registered Dietician (RD)**—The highest level of nutritionist who has earned a bachelor's degree in nutrition and passed a board exam, these specialists focus on helping patients identify their specific nutrition needs based on a range of individual factors.

**Wellness Centers**—Health centers where one can find a variety of health and fitness professionals, including exercise physiologists, registered dietitians, nurse practitioners, MDs, DOs, and more. Some offer a variety of services from yoga and meditation to screening for proper movement and taking blood work to check vitamin and hormone levels and putting together an intuitive nutrition program for an individual's specific needs.

CPSIA information can be obtained
at www.ICGtesting.com
Printed in the USA
BVHW051234131221
623913BV00011B/504/J